What if
it really is...?

Even if we'd rather not find the answer in the mind,
would it be worth having a look there,
just in case?

Mary Ratcliffe

Grosvenor House
Publishing Limited

Mary Ratcliffe is hereby identified as author of this
work in accordance with Section 77 of the Copyright, Designs
and Patents Act 1988

The book cover picture is copyright to ©Andrea Danti/Fotolia

This book is published by
Grosvenor House Publishing Ltd
28-30 High Street, Guildford, Surrey, GU1 3HY.
www.grosvenorhousepublishing.co.uk

Lesserian Curative Hypnotherapy™ and
LCH® are registered trademarks and
use of them is subject to UK law.

A CIP record for this book
is available from the British Library

ISBN 978-1-907211-45-4

For Michael

Reviews

Mary has used a series of (often humorous) conversations to methodically explain the premises that form the foundations of Lesserian Curative Hypnotherapy (LCH). This book provides an accessible introduction to people wishing to find out more about LCH but is also an essential read for practitioners that builds on the work of the founder of Curative Hypnotherapy, David Lesser, and his two original texts. The simplicity of the writing style belies the complexity of the issues discussed. There is an old Chinese proverb that says, 'A single conversation with a wise person is worth a month's study of books'. This book gives you three things – wisdom, good conversation and a good read.

Farrukh Akhtar - Senior Lecturer in Social Work, Kingston University

%%%

WHAT IF IT REALLY IS...? is a great introduction and explanation of the fascinating world of LCH and the possibly even more fascinating world of our subconscious mind. Whether you are seeking treatment, considering embarking on a career in LCH, already involved with Hypnotherapy, or simply interested in the potential power of your own subconscious this book is invaluable... an absolute 'must have'....

Mary explains in her own unique way, her experiences and understanding of the subconscious and its capabilities, based on her work in LCH to date and her own personal journey through treatment , writing with clarity and conviction not to mention humour, on a subject which has the possibility of changing people's lives for the better.

Peppered with real 'penny-dropping' moments, this book is an essential bit of kit....don't leave home without it!

Jo Baldwin - Hypnotherapist

%%%

I thoroughly enjoyed it, thank you. It makes a difficult subject accessible, the format made it palatable and your big finish (your personal story) was an amazing testament.

It satisfied me on two levels a) as a potential therapist b) as a potential patient and it was enough to make me feel hooked.

Angie Broad M.A. Theatre Studies

%%%

Is there an unconscious mind that controls much of what we do, not always in ways that we like? Why do we do what we do and can we take control and change it? These have been burning and unanswered questions for many of us. With powerful use of illustration and metaphor, the author provides the most convincing evidence yet that a part of our mind is in control of our behaviour and that we can access that part and change what we do. Using every day events, this book is full of examples that you will recognise in yourself. Compelling, thought provoking and full of insight. This book will resonate with your soul.

Harry Parker BSc (Hons) Behavioural Sciences

Contents

CONTENTS

Foreword

The greater the understanding of how something works; the more effectively we can use and apply that knowledge. The more diverse and varied the explanations from differing perspectives; the greater our understanding of that subject and the easier it is to spread and share it amongst others.

So, when Mary Ratcliffe first approached me to ask how I would feel about her writing a book about LCH® treatment, there was only one reason why I did not bite her hand off.... I knew she would type faster with it!

The following pages are Mary's views, her opinions, her understanding and all explained in Mary's own unique and gentle way. However, her descriptions and explanations accurately portray the extent to which we now understand how the subconscious works; how we can work together with it in order to achieve tremendous benefits for others.

It has been more than 20 years since the late David Lesser wrote the first two books about Curative Hypnotherapy (Hypnotherapy Explained: 1985 & The Book of Hypnosis: 1989) and to date, they remain the only two books available on the subject. Across those years, working in my own practice and learning from my own students on the courses, my understanding and the application of Curative Hypnotherapy grew and steadily evolved into what is now called LCH®.

All this work over all this time – analysing, de-constructing, scrutinising, testing, expanding, revising and then dissecting and examining again what I had learnt - Mary has managed to distil succinctly into this publication in a beautifully simple and straightforward way. Because of these immense advancements since those first two books were published, a new book is long overdue - and my gratitude goes to Mary for doing such a sterling job.

My hope is that this book will inspire you to find out more, to seek out other explanations, to ask questions, to look for proof – but if nothing else, I hope, (through Mary's eyes) you will simply enjoy looking at the world from a slightly different perspective.

Helen Lesser

Principal: Therapy Training College, Birmingham. 2010.

Acknowledgements

Various people have helped in various ways, with ideas, support, encouragement and seemingly endless patience.

Apologies that I haven't been able to include everyone by name, but many thanks to all those who have listened to my ramblings and humoured me so good-naturedly as I've gone off on some latest idea – and special thanks to those who have valiantly stayed awake and even more for those who have bravely offered some comment or question that invariably set me off yet again with another full tank of fuel.

A huge thank-you to Helen Lesser, Michael Cardis, Farrukh Akhtar, Tara Culhane-Lock, Angie Broad, Vanita Grad, Gwen Blundell, Harry Parker, Jo Baldwin. Katrina Steedman, Tracie Jarvis, Garry Hart, Hannah and Tim Dolmansley, who have done all of the above and also read various drafts along the way. They have offered constructive comments and supplied enough enthusiasm to keep me going when, from time to time, my own energy and self-confidence took a dive.

Clearly none of this would have been possible without Lesserian Curative Hypnotherapy (LCH) being invented and refined by David and Helen Lesser.

If the style of the book is not totally infuriating, then we have Farrukh to thank for her honesty and her inspired suggestions for improvement.

And if, in a senior moment, I've missed a name or two here, apologies for that and please know that all the help I've received has always been much appreciated and has contributed to the completion of this book, which has been, for me, an epic endeavour.

All in the mind?

There's been a great deal of discussion over the years about the descriptive terms 'psychosomatic' and 'all in the mind' - and of how they come across to us, particularly if our state of health is ever described in that way. It feels preferable in some way to have a physical rather than a psychological condition. Our state of illness, our lack of health seems to be validated by being scientifically measurable, detectable by a blood test, an X-ray or an MRI scan.

It can feel better once we get a diagnosis. People can doubt that we're ill if they only have our word for it that we have some pain, fatigue or exhaustion, lack of mobility, some strange sensory experience like ringing in the ears or whatever – and all the tests prove negative. And this can be a cause for more concern if we find ourselves so debilitated that we are unable to work or study. And there's even more to worry about if those symptoms are becoming steadily more severe, even more frequent.

So if we hear the expression, 'it's all in the mind', we can perceive it as negative - a criticism that is condescending and insulting. If we have a physical illness but the tests prove inconclusive, we might wonder if that signifies that it's psychological or psychosomatic. We can assume we're being told to 'get over it', to 'pull ourselves together', that it's not real – that it only exists in our imagination. And yet our symptoms, whether physical or psychological, are very real, uncomfortable, painful or even agonising, and certainly worrying. So such messages can be most unwelcome!

And conversely, if an illness or condition is clearly visible to the various tests employed by medical science, does that necessarily mean that it isn't 'all in the mind'? If there is a detectable change in a blood chemical or the functioning of an organ such as the liver or kidney, what caused that? Maybe it was some external factor that caused it, but in most cases, we would expect that factor to cause the same change in everyone in the vicinity – and in most cases, it doesn't. And does anything happen for no reason at all – just by chance – some purely random phenomenon?

So much of the medical, clinical research that is constantly being carried out is getting amazing results in the fields of cancer, heart disease, AIDS, diabetes, spinal injury, plastic surgery. Many more illnesses and traumas can now be recovered from. People are able to survive and live happy and productive lives after a diagnosis that was previously considered a prison sentence - or even a death sentence.

Consider the painstaking and diligent work of many doctors and scientists collaborating on their combined aim of the health and comfort of sick and injured people. They examine the contents of test-tubes, put slides under microscopes and wait patiently for results to develop from what is growing in a culture dish. Then the news breaks. Someone has found another gene for this, another antidote for that and we sigh with relief as yet another illness becomes measurable, quantifiable and therefore diagnosable and correctable.

But there are some illnesses and diseases that are still popularly regarded as incurable. We can understand people questioning why, with all the money and science and research, all the best brains in the world working towards the health of us all, why we aren't as healthy as was predicted when our great health service was first invented.

Some drugs and other medical interventions show such promising results initially, and seem like a total cure-all when first licensed, but later emerge as a solution for only a handful of special cases. Some drugs continue to achieve all the benefits they were designed for, but only at the cost of side-effects that are, in some cases, only marginally less severe than the illnesses they have halted.

Many people live with all kinds of long-term, debilitating symptoms and conditions, physical and psychological, having had all the treatment deemed appropriate based on the very best of scientific research and testing of whatever their state of health is displaying to them and to their specialists. Either nothing has worked, or it worked for a while, but long-term, the condition itself remains to get in the way of the happy, healthy and productive life that seemed to be stretching ahead of them before this descent into pain, immobility, fear and worry.

People learn to live with their illness, manage their symptoms, control their discomfort and pain, because the people who have devoted their lives to the cause of health and wellbeing have used all the tools in their toolbox and can now only offer palliative care and a hope that those researchers will soon find a cure.

So if more success and more progress are needed, how about asking some different questions? If the questions we've been asking up to now haven't brought as much health as we hoped and expected, would it be worth looking at it all from a completely different angle?

And as we seem to prefer to learn that it's physical rather than psychological, it seems that we tend to fund similar kinds of physical scientific research.

Even if we'd all rather not find the answer in the mind, would it be worth having a look there, just in case?

What if 'it's all in the mind' means that, actually, there's another avenue we haven't explored quite so fully yet. What if it's more liberating than condescending, full of possibilities and potential rather than frustration and hopelessness? What if 'the mind' that it's 'all in' is a part that is hidden from us? And what if, in that hidden part of the mind, there is an, as yet, barely explored vital link in the chain of that illness/wellness spectrum that we all inhabit?

If a physical illness or condition is caused by a raised level of some blood chemical or a reduced or impaired functioning of some vital organ, why did that happen? Could a thought, chosen or uninvited, have triggered that change? Could some subconscious processing have set up some kind of chain reaction that resulted in some disease or syndrome?

If that seems like a bizarre proposition, and if you're wondering what could have generated such questions....

If you want to consider some different ideas, look at things from an angle that you've maybe not seen in exactly this way before....

If you have an illness or condition that you are managing, living with – giving time each day to measures that minimise its effects - and wonder if there's something out there that can help you to fully resolve it, so you can get on with your life in the way that you want to....

If you are looking at various forms of therapy because you are considering training to be a therapist and don't know yet which direction is best for you.....

If you are reading purely out of interest, not sure where this will take you, and hoping to enjoy the journey, to stimulate your enquiring mind, to learn something that might help in shedding some light on any current dilemmas or paradoxes....

You might want to know that my journey of discovery hasn't been conducted in any laboratory. It's taken place mainly as a result of my observations, my own study, of life in general, mine and those around me, and of my training and work as a therapist, working with that intriguing and fascinating creature, the subconscious mind.

And I'm not the only one to ask some of these questions.

Apart from the personal information about me, and all the detail about treatment I've received, no individual piece of information can be relied on to be factual. It's all mixed up and anonymised, based on various people, their conversations with me, my observations of them when I was people-watching, and from treatments I have given and received.

Two of my friends

My friend Pat is looking for a career change and is short of ideas. My friend Chris is living with various uncomfortable symptoms and issues - has had all sorts of tests and treatments that have brought some relief but not enough - and is beginning to consider the world of complementary and alternative medicine.

Pat and I met up for a coffee. We're old friends but we'd lost touch and haven't actually seen each other for many years. I offered a few details about my career path over the last few years and Pat began to take a keener interest, to ask some questions that set me off. It doesn't take much - as many friends, loads of acquaintances, and even total strangers have learnt to their cost from time to time.

I explained that the kind of hypnotherapy that I trained in is different from many other kinds of hypnotherapy and that those differences can lead and have led to the mysterious disappearance of real and detectable physical conditions and symptoms. I trained in Lesserian Curative Hypnotherapy (LCH) and as far as I know, nothing like it exists anywhere! A huge statement – but if it did exist somewhere, I feel sure I would have heard of it. It's something to shout from the rooftops about because its potential and actual benefits are so great that it will be a crying shame if it isn't fully examined and investigated and replicated for the benefit of people in any way less healthy and/or less happy that they would like to be.

It's very new, in the great scheme of things, but it is growing steadily. LCH therapists are working tirelessly towards improving their own and our collective clinical results. Some of those therapists are also working towards developing the way it is taught and developed for students and newly qualified therapists.

So it was no surprise to me that Pat had never heard of it. We started mulling over some of the ideas, concepts, theories and hypotheses, and the result was something along the lines of the following.

Me: What is the brain?

Pat: *It's an organ in the body, part of the central nervous system, and it controls other organs and systems and movements.*

Me: What is the mind?

Pat: *It's what we think with. It's our awareness, our consciousness.*

Me: And is it a physical thing like the brain?

Pat: *No I don't think it is.*

Me: So can we detect it directly in any way?

Pat: *No I don't think so.*

Me: So how can we learn about it?

Pat: *By studying behaviour, making psychological theories and then testing them out on humans to see if they behave as we predict.*

Me: And does the mind control anything other than behaviour?

Pat: *Yes. It's responsible for thoughts, feelings and emotions.*

Me: And what about those thoughts, feelings and emotions that we don't want but can't get rid of using willpower?

Pat: *They must come from the subconscious mind.*

Me: So there's another part of the mind that we call subconscious and we need to study that part as well, but as it's hidden from our consciousness, again, how can we learn about it?

Pat: *Again, by making theories and testing them out.*

Me: If we can't see or detect the mind in any way, just observe the results of the action of the mind, can we start by simply defining the mind as being what controls us?

Pat: *Yes, ok.*

Me: And can we simply split the mind into 2 areas, the conscious part and the subconscious part?

Pat: *Yes.*

Me: So if the conscious part is the part we are aware of, the thinking, analysing, choosing, deciding part, then everything else, everything outside of our awareness or control is the subconscious part. Is that a workable definition?

Pat: *Again, yes.*

Me: So how about starting by deciding which bits of our mind control which parts of us?

Pat: *Ok*

Me: Is the digestive system consciously or subconsciously controlled?

Pat: *Subconsciously.*

Me: What about the breathing?

Pat: *It's both. It goes on when we're not thinking about it and when we're asleep, but we can override it up to a point.*

Me: So I can hold my breath?

Pat: *Yes for a while.*

Me: What happens if I decide or choose to hold my breath for 10 minutes?

Pat: *You'd eventually collapse and become unconscious.*

Me: And what happens to my breathing then?

Pat: *It starts up again.*

Me: So something has overridden my willpower and caused my breathing to start again, is that right?

Pat: *Yes.*

Me: So what did that?

Pat: *The subconscious mind.*

Me: Why would it do that?

Pat: *To keep us alive.*

Me: So is it a kind of life-support system?

Pat: *Yes.*

Me: And what about blinking?

Pat: *It's the same as breathing. It happens automatically but we can override it.*

Me: And if I try to override it by keeping my eyes open constantly for an hour, what happens?

Pat: *It becomes really painful and eventually the pain forces you to blink.*

Me: And again, what did that?

Pat: *The subconscious mind.*

Me: And why?

Pat: *Because the surface of the eye needs to stay clean and moist in order to function well. If it dried out, then the process of closing the eyes to sleep would cause friction and damage their surface.*

Me: So it's not just keeping me alive, it's keeping me healthy too, keeping things working well, is that right?

Pat: *Yes.*

Me: Is picking up a pencil a conscious or subconscious act?

Pat: *It's conscious.*

Me: How many muscles does it take to pick up a pencil?

Pat: *I don't know.*

Me: What does it take to make a hand or an arm or a leg move?

Pat: *Various muscles have to contract and relax in pairs.*

Me: What causes a muscle to relax?

Pat: *I don't know. I think that's its default state.*

Me: What causes a muscle to contract?

Pat: *The brain sends an impulse down a nerve which causes the muscle contraction.*

Me: What tells the brain to send that particular impulse at that time?

Pat: *The mind.*

Me: And if you don't consciously know even how many muscles it takes to pick up a pencil, never mind how much each needs to move, are you able to give those instructions consciously?

Pat: *No.*

Me: So which part of the mind gave those instructions?

Pat: *The subconscious part.*

Me: Ok, so is picking up a pencil a conscious or subconscious act?

Pat: *I'm still not sure. I decided to pick it up, so that part is conscious.*

Me: So might it be a combination of conscious intention and subconsciously-determined detailed instructions?

Pat: *Yes, that sounds likely.*

Me: And could it ever be purely subconscious?

Pat: *No – there always has to be a conscious intention.*

Me: Do you ever move your hands around when you speak?

Pat: *Yes*

Me: Do you choose to do that?

Pat: *Yes, I do it to emphasise or illustrate a point.*

Me: To the person you are talking to?

Pat: *Yes*

Me: And have you ever found yourself moving your hands around to emphasise or illustrate a point when you're alone and talking to someone on the phone?

Pat: *Yes.*

Me: Why do you do that?

Pat: *I don't know.*

Me: Did you choose to?

Pat: *No, I guess it's just a habit.*

Me: And as it takes instructions from the mind to make your hands move, and you didn't give those instructions intentionally, you didn't even intend to move your hands when talking on the phone, which part of your mind gave the instructions?

Pat: *The subconscious part.*

Me: So could a movement of your hand be purely a subconscious act?

Pat: *Ok, I'll go for that – yes it could be.*

Me: And what about driving – is that conscious or subconscious?

Pat: *I suppose it should be conscious but I think we all drive on autopilot at least some of the time.*

Me: And when we're on autopilot, do we still react automatically and appropriately to an emergency by slamming on the brakes or swerving or whatever is the best option?

Pat: *Yes*

Me: And if there's no emergency, do we still keep a safe distance from the car in front?

Pat: *Yes*

Me: So when we're on autopilot, do we tend to drive safely?

Pat: *Yes*

Me: And the subconscious keeps us safe even when we're distracted by the radio or a daydream or a conversation with a passenger, is that right?

Pat: *Yes.*

Me: What creates habits?

Pat: *The conscious mind starts it off because I choose to do something, then I do it often enough that it becomes automatic. The subconscious mind takes over at that point.*

Me: I agree. And it's a very important process. We could never do anything even slightly complex without that habit or automatic mechanism. We couldn't drive a car, something many people take for granted after some months or years of practice, if things didn't become automatic as we learnt. The driving instructor has to give loads of instructions on that first lesson to get us to set off, drive a short distance and then stop again. Engine started, press the clutch, (that's the pedal on the left), hand on gear lever, engage first gear (that's the one in the top left hand corner), now check your mirror, look over your shoulder to check there's nothing in your blind-spot, foot on the accelerator (that's the pedal on the right)... and we haven't even moved yet.

So habits are vital to our ability to live our lives.

But sometimes those habits need to change. We have been driving in the UK for years and never give it a thought now. We've set off without being aware of any of those actions because something on the radio has set us off on some train of thought. Then we go to the continent on holiday and hire a car. The steering wheel is on the other side. At first, so much is unfamiliar that we think it all through. The gear lever is on the other side. We need to drive on the other side of the road. There's no way, on that first continental driving experience, that we could let our attention focus on the radio. We'd probably never even think to turn it on.

Then, after a few driving experiences, we start to get the hang of it and relax a bit. That's when those automatic habits come back in and trip us up. We go for the gear lever and find ourselves hitting our hand against the door. We set off on a quiet road with no other traffic on the move, and start travelling on the left hand side until we notice and quickly correct ourselves.

But by the end of the holiday, those habits have adjusted to our new environment and we can relax and drive effectively after only a week of re-training. And when we get back home, we need a little concentration at first, but it's not that long before the automatic left-hand-drive habits take over again.

And what's doing all that?

Pat: *The subconscious mind.*

Me: Yes. It responds to the new circumstances, to our changed intentions, by changing the automatic responses. So what about a habit we chose in the past but now want to change? It could be smoking, excessive alcohol, some other drug,

1 6

shopping, gambling, excessive eating. So if we consciously choose to give up because of the effects it's having on our health, our finances, our relationships, because it takes over and makes us feel out of control, why don't those habits change?

Pat: *Some of those are addictive substances.*

Me: Could someone be addicted to alcohol, cigarettes and sleeping tablets all at the same time?

Pat: *Yes. Lots of people are.*

Me: And might they be able to break their addiction to sleeping tablets using willpower?

Pat: *Yes, they might. I think some people have.*

Me: So even though it's an addictive substance, some people have broken the habit using willpower?

Pat: *Yes*

Me: And someone who only has that one addiction, to sleeping tablets, might they be unable to break that addiction using willpower?

Pat: *Yes. There are many people who can't break that addiction without professional help.*

Me: So if one person can break their sleeping tablet addiction but someone else can't, what explains that difference?

Pat: *Maybe they need something, a support, a crutch. Maybe they can manage if they have at least one. And maybe they smoke and drink more to compensate.*

Me: So if a substance can be addictive but we can break that if we have another substance to take its place, what explains that?

Pat: *They have an addictive personality.*

Me: And would someone with that kind of personality find that all habits were out of their control? Would they find themselves unable to adapt to driving on the continent?

Pat: *No, but that's a different kind of habit. It's nothing to do with a need for support.*

Me: And if someone has an addictive personality, were they born with it? Is it nature or nurture?

Pat: *I don't know. Maybe it's a combination of the two.*

Me: Some people believe that there's no cure, so that, for example, an alcoholic is always an alcoholic. There's a common acceptance that we would have to completely abstain from alcohol for the rest of our life if we ever developed severe alcohol dependence. We would need to take one day at a time and avoid all situations that could trip us up. We wouldn't even be able to risk a mouthful of Aunty Peggy's trifle in case she forgot and put in a spoonful of sherry. People believe that because that has been the experience of most people up to now.

And many people see cigarette smoking the same way – that the ex-smoker is harbouring a dormant virus, waiting to leap up and take hold again if they ever so much as take a drag of a cigarette in order to light it for a friend.

But if the subconscious mind is in control of all habits, and an addiction is a kind of habit, and it isn't about the substance itself, more about the person's need for something, like support, then has anyone actually asked the subconscious mind why it's maintaining that habit or addiction or that need for support?

Pat: *I don't know.*

Me: Well if they haven't, would it be worth asking?

Pat: *Of course, but how would you be able to do that?*

The placebo effect

Pat has seen some of the logic and is intrigued.

Pat: *Does the subconscious mind make us ill, then? It doesn't seem to make sense to me. Does it create illnesses and then fix them? We've agreed that it controls the digestive system, so could it be responsible for malfunctions in that area?*

Me: Let's think about the placebo effect – see if that can help us understand more. How does the placebo effect work?

Pat: *I don't know.*

Me: We know it does work because it plays a part in every modern-day drug trial. In such experiments, some people get better with no intervention because of the well-known capability of the human body to fight illnesses and diseases, to mend broken bones, to heal wounds, to restore health and balance without any external intervention other than to create a conducive environment such as good nutrition and cleanliness.

In most cases, even more people get better because they were given a therapeutic intervention, e.g. a form of medication containing a chemical combination designed to correct some detected

imbalance in the body of the sick person –
something to restore balance and correct
functioning to an organ or system within the
body.

But usually, somewhere between the percentage
who benefit from the body's own mechanisms and
those who recover as a result of that researched
and scientifically well-founded medicine, is a
group whose condition improves because they
were given a tablet and told it might contain the
drug being tested.

As far as my amateur understanding goes, a higher
proportion of people in these tests recover when
given an inactive pill they thought might be active
and beneficial, than recovered without that pill.

Pat: *That's a bit complicated! Can you give me an
example?*

Me: 300 people have illness xyz. 100 of them (group A)
receive no medical treatment of any kind. Another
hundred (group B) are treated exactly the same
except that they take a totally inert pill once a day
and are told they are taking part in a clinical trial
for a new drug that has performed extremely well
in lab tests. We don't need to concern ourselves
right now with the 100 that got the medicine being
tested, (group C).

35 of group A recover. 50 of group B recover.

Assuming no other factors skew the results in any
way, they are of similar ages and backgrounds and
general health, then we could predict that 35 of

group B would have recovered without the pill. If we do many tests, and we get pretty close to Group A 35% and Group B 50% recoveries from all those tests, then we can argue that 15 of those people recovered purely from being given a totally inert substance and being told that it might be beneficial.

We know loads about the many correcting and balancing systems in the body. When we have a small cut, we bleed, it scabs over. The scab keeps out infection and allows the skin to heal. If we pick off that scab, it might bleed again, scab over again and begin to heal again. If left in place, the scab will stay there until the skin underneath is strong enough to cope without the scab, at which time it falls off all on its own.

If we have a big cut, a scab can't form because of the flowing blood, and if we don't restrict that flow soon enough, we could lose so much blood that our brain and other vital organs are at risk of being damaged because of the lack of blood, oxygen and nutrients. We feel faint, we lie down, our blood pressure falls. All of that buys us some time and increases our chances of surviving by reducing the rate of blood loss and assisting in the flow of blood to the brain because the heart doesn't have to work so hard against gravity to send it there.

If we caught some specific childhood illnesses when we were very young, then we probably gained enough immunity to protect us from suffering the same illnesses later in life. The immune system has enough information, has developed the antibodies, so that any repeat contact with the same infection, bacteria or virus is fought and dispatched – often before any outward sign of the illness has chance to appear.

All of these, and many more, just happen automatically. It's how we're made. We have the most fantastic design that arrives with the basic software to deal with all that was around when our parents were growing up – and with the learning capability to adapt, given enough time, to any new pathogens.

Pat: *So what is going on with the placebo?*

If there's nothing except the thought that I've been given, or might have been given, a magic pill or potion to cause that significant improvement in my condition, then did that thought itself cause me to heal, or to heal more quickly? Are all those wonderful healing and balancing systems connected in some way to my conscious mind? Is it the thought, is it the intention, is it the belief or trust in the doctor, the researcher, is it the assumption that I've been given a cure? Is it the conscious mind or the subconscious mind – or a combination of both, that is contributing to this strange and wonderful benefit?

Me: If my body reacts badly to a certain type of food for some reason, e.g. if the presence of some component in that food in my digestive system would cause damage to some major organ, then the best thing the body's healing processes could do for me would be to get rid of that component rapidly, before it has chance to reach that organ. The quickest way to do that would be to induce vomiting.

If that potential damage were so severe, even life-threatening, then even if there were only the slightest possibility that what I had eaten might have contained that component, then it wouldn't make sense to wait for my internal laboratory to get back with the results – if it could kill me if it reached my liver, then it's a much lesser evil to induce vomiting that might turn out afterwards not to have actually been required.

So if my body systems detect that component, then the best action my body can take is to get rid of the whole batch, give it a good rinse round, and keep going until all traces of the entire contents of the digestive system have been well washed away.

Something could cause me to suspect that I may have eaten something containing something harmful to me. I might then feel very ill, and as unpleasant as it is, and as much as I resist that ordeal, it happens anyway. My body gets rid of that food rapidly and totally, in spite of my wish not to. I may then learn afterwards that there was nothing in that meal that would have caused me any harm.

And the body systems that can detect a certain kind of food or some bacteria or poison within it,

I believe these are all controlled by the subconscious mind. And clearly the thought that I might have eaten something dodgy, that's a product of the conscious mind.

Pat: *One way or another, we keep coming back to the mind causing things to happen to the body. What is going on?*

What if...

Pat: *I'm just getting more and more puzzled. Do you have an example that explains it?*

Me: Fiona has angina. She gets pain when she exerts herself. She takes her medication when the pain comes on and tries to keep herself away from physical and psychological stress.

But the cause of the angina is the furred up arteries, the plaque that is lining the walls of her blood vessels so that the extra blood flow needed at certain times hasn't got enough room to flow freely. The pipes are now too narrow. So the medical team do a kind of pipe-cleaning process to clear the debris away – the debris from many years of a rich diet, an inactive lifestyle and a short mental fuse. Fiona, my imaginary angina-sufferer is highly strung.

She now has clean, clear arteries and the blood flow can increase when necessary, but she still has the same diet and is just as nervy, just as unfit and inactive as before – so steadily, the deposits return.

Her medical team give her all the information and persuasion to make the appropriate lifestyle changes. She sees the logic, understands the process, and she makes some changes. She works hard at it, and for a while, she succeeds. But this isn't a one-off fix – she needs this new lifestyle for the rest of her life – and it's hard work. It doesn't come naturally.

It's as if she needs to fight against her nature.

She reacts to the highs and lows of life and work and family by a combination of growling at anyone who gets in her way and self-medicating with whatever seems most appropriate or appealing in her medicine cabinet – chocolate, crisps, wine, lager, a take-away...

If treatment stops short here with a message from the doctor that she needs to get herself and her life in order, then with that habitual way of coping with life, she has very little chance of turning it around and creating healthier habits.

Pat: *Yes I agree. So what can be done – and how can she be helped. Is something causing her to prefer those particular forms of food and alcohol self-medication?*

Me: We could describe it as another layer. There's something underneath – something causing that short fuse which in turn causes the heightened emotions that are so uncomfortable and need to be calmed by a Danish pastry and a cream-topped hot chocolate.

Pat: *What about when someone has an illness and the medical team successfully treat it. It's completely cured. But then they develop another illness. The same happens again. I know of a few people like that, where they just seem to suffer one thing after another. There's always a cure – but then another illness comes along. If someone is serially ill, just one thing after another, could that be because there's another layer? Is there sometimes a need to be ill?*

Me: Yes – and the illness doesn't need to be a specific one, sometimes any will do. Maybe it just needs to be of a certain seriousness or intensity. So the medical interventions are successful, but the need for some kind of illness, some kind of symptom hasn't been considered and hasn't been targeted.

Pat: *If such a need were to exist, would that also explain the situations where the illness is cured but from time to time, relapses occur? The illness could disappear for a period of time and then come back. There are lots of illnesses where that happens. There are also some people who recover fully from the same types of illnesses that other people find just keep coming back again and again. Might that be because there is an as yet unresolved need to be ill?*

Me: Yes – all of those types of situations could be explained by another, deeper layer, an underlying cause.

Pat: *And what about when someone lives for many years in an unhappy marriage, a nightmare job or career, then finds that life has taken a turn for the better. The marriage could have ended by widowhood or*

*divorce and been followed by a calm and happy
state as a singleton, or a warm and loving new
relationship. The job could have been lost through
redundancy and replaced by a challenging and
fulfilling move into self-employment.*

*Then, just as life looks like it's finally got a chance
of being happy, some serious, debilitating, life-
threatening condition takes over and turns it all
sour. I've heard of quite a few examples like that,
and I even know one or two affected that way.
Could there be an underlying need to suffer?
And if there were such a need, would that explain
this pattern?*

Me: I think you're getting the hang of this. Fancy
writing a book about it?

When someone has an accident while driving, if it's
assessed as having been a result of their carelessness
or even recklessness behind the wheel, then they
will be given the appropriate punishment. But if it
was caused by a momentary loss of concentration,
and resulted in the death or permanent disability of
the driver's loved one, then the court will often issue
a suspended sentence in recognition that the driver
is already being severely punished far beyond
appropriateness based on their intention and
overall level of care.

Pat: *So could there be something similar going on here?
Could there be some deep, subconscious belief in
a need or deserving of some punishment that is
being met by the nightmare home and work life?
And if that nightmare were to end, then would the*

'Court' need to step in and introduce some
punishment of its own, some illness, some disability,
some strange undiagnosable pain, some worryingly
deteriorating and debilitating condition? Does that
kind of thing happen? And if so, could that 'other
layer' explain it? And if so, what do we do about it?

Me: Yes it could explain it, but we need a lot more to
go on before we're anywhere near fixing it.

Pat: *Surely you can't fix anything that's genetic or*
hereditary though, can you?

Me: When scientists study samples in a laboratory,
they take them out of the person's body and
examine them under a microscope. But maybe
that tiny piece of tissue or drop of blood or
fragment of bone behaves differently now that it
has been removed from the body, from the central
nervous system, from the mind. A vast quantity of
research is done into genes, into whether sufferers
of specific diseases have any genes in common.

Pat: *Yes, I can't remember the details but there's*
research that has shown people with disease X
also have gene A – so are those people stuck with
their illnesses, or are they going to be fixed when
gene therapy finds the specific cure for disease X?

Me: Yes but what about those few annoying
exceptions, those few people who have disease X
and don't have gene A, and those people who
have gene A but don't have disease X.

Pat: *Well they imply that if you have that gene, then you*
WILL get that illness. You just haven't got it yet.

You have a ticking time bomb inside you. And those that have the disease but not the gene, maybe they have a variant of the disease caused by a different gene that hasn't been identified yet.

Me: Yes that's all true – that could explain it, but another type of research is looking more into whether the gene is switched on or off. And if that testing is done outside the body, or even at a different time, the gene could be off when it was previously on, or vice versa.

I have various pieces of electrical equipment with, broadly, 2 different types of switches, hard ones and soft ones. If I switch my hairdryer on using the switch on its handle, and then unplug it from the mains, it's plain to see that it's still set to 'ON'. If I plug it in again, it will start up again. It had stayed in the 'ON' position. If I do the same kind of thing with my kettle, the switch reverts to 'OFF' as soon as the power is removed. If I plug it back in, it stays off until I switch it back on.

Pat: *So are genes like switches, and if so, which kind of switches are they like? Do they stay in the same state as they were when 'unplugged' or do they always revert to 'OFF'?*

Me: As far as I understand, there's plenty of research in this area, but as I'm not a scientist and I haven't studied it, I don't have any sources to quote. Other than finding myself vaguely aware of it, I can't add any kind of evidence. I'm simply saying that that's another plausible theory or possible explanation of some of the findings.

If there's a gene that is implicated in a particular disease, but at least one sufferer of the disease doesn't have that gene, and/or, at least one person who doesn't have the disease does have the gene, then it's possibly less about the existence of the gene than whether or not the gene is active.

Pat: *And could the ON/OFF state of the gene be driven by the mind, by the conscious mind, by a thought, by the subconscious mind, by a belief?*

Me: Well I believe it could and have a vague recollection of hearing or reading of scientific findings that seem to support that idea.

The subconscious mind

Pat: *I've started thinking more about the subconscious mind, but it's really just words to me. I don't really have any idea of what it is or what it's like. It fascinates me and intrigues me. Have you got some way of helping me get more of an understanding of what it is, what it does, what it's capable of doing, and why it does what it does?*

Me: Would it help if I describe it as a person and try to predict what kind of person it might be?

Pat: *Yes, I'm sure that would help.*

Me: Ok. We can start with – the subconscious mind as our personal assistant. Have you ever found yourself suddenly remembering someone's birthday or anniversary?

Pat: *Yes of course.*

Me: Who reminded you?

Pat: *If I had a personal assistant, they would do it, so ok – I'm with you so far.*

Me: Have you ever been standing in a crowded room talking happily to someone nearby, hardly aware of the hum of conversation around you, and then suddenly you notice that someone at the other side of the room has just said your name?

Pat: *Again yes.*

Me: Who nudged you?

Pat: *Ok, I'm happy this has some potential. Carry on.*

Me: If you ever leave the house with your mind totally on where you are going and your plans for the day and then wonder if you locked the door, then I'm confident that you found, on checking, that it's nearly always locked.

If you regularly drive your normal route to work and get there with hardly a thought about the journey, the fact that you're sitting here with me now means your personal assistant is a very safe driver.

What about a normal day, totally engrossed in work or play, but regularly, several times a day, you get hungry and get a strong urge to eat. And it's normally about the same times each day, the time when the canteen is open or when today's scones have just arrived.

On the other hand, what if there's some emergency going on, if some family member needs urgent medical attention and reassurance? You take them to A&E and hold their hand til their injury is treated – and then, spookily, along with that sense of relief, suddenly you notice that you haven't eaten for 8 hours – and could do with some food – now!

The subconscious does all these things – and if you were to note down all it does, you'd end up with a very long list, the kind of list that most of us share, and this gives me enough justification to describe the subconscious mind as a personal assistant.

Pat: *Yes it helps me understand a bit more.*

Me: And it also helps me to work with this mysterious, hidden part of the mind, to predict what it might do, and in my clinical practice, to find ways to help it resolve issues.

Pat: *Ok – so how does this help a guy who wants to stop smoking, wants to get a good night's sleep or needs to lose some weight?*

Me: Personal assistants can sometimes get it wrong. However good they are, fantastic and efficient, they might just let us down. Maybe they do everything else perfectly, but there's just one thing they do wrong and we don't know why.

Maybe this guy's personal assistant just keeps lighting him another cigarette, handing him another can of lager or bar of chocolate when he hadn't given it a thought and didn't really want one.

And maybe the assistant keeps him awake at night with endless chatter about things that could wait until the morning.

Pat: *And the spider phobic. What's his assistant up to?*

Me: Maybe he's being ultra careful, covering his back and taking no chances, insisting that that harmless domestic money spider must be treated as if it's actually as dangerous as a tarantula until proved otherwise.

Pat: *And someone that's suffering from anxiety or panic attacks?*

Me: Maybe his assistant does everything exactly as he wants them to, but they keep asking for reassurance, wondering if they're doing ok, expecting that they must be doing something wrong.

Pat: *And how does that help with treatment?*

Me: Maybe there was something that he told them years ago – something he's forgotten about but they haven't – something that is now just one small entry in that huge instruction manual that they've been building up since the day he was born, something that needs reviewing and maybe updating.

Pat: *And is that what you do in your clinical practice?*

Me: Yes, that's where LCH comes in. This technique, and all the understanding behind it, can work with that personal assistant and help him or her find and fix whatever it is that has got in the way of that wonderful employee being totally, without exception, the best we could wish for.

What is LCH?

Pat: *So what is LCH?*

Me: It stands for Lesserian Curative Hypnotherapy.
It's called Lesserian because it was invented and
refined by David Lesser and his daughter, Helen.

LCH is a form of therapy that works with the
subconscious mind to find and help resolve the
underlying cause or need for any consciously
unwanted symptom, condition or issue.

With LCH theory and understanding, it makes
as much sense to work directly on the presenting
problem as it does to say: -

'That fire alarm is making a very annoying noise
so I'll just switch it off. Oh that's a relief. I can go
back to reading my book now.'

Or even: -

'The smoke alarm had gone off because of all that
smoke. I know, I'll open that door and window, get a
good blast of fresh air through here and clear out all
that smoke. Oh great, the smoke alarm has stopped
now. Now I can go back to my afternoon nap.'

Or even: -

'That smoke alarm means something needs attention. The toaster is plugged in but the switch is off, and yet it's smoking. No worries. I'll just unplug it from the wall. It's safe now. I'll just finish my packing and get off to the station. Mum and Dad will be here for the weekend so they can feed the cat while I'm away'.

Pat: *Scary!!!*

Me: Yes I agree and that's why I won't rest until I feel like my verdict is safe, until it makes sense – and the symptom has gone away. I might be happy if I found that my patient's toaster had a loose wire in the plug, that it had been fitted by her son when he was a teenager and liked doing DIY most after a trip to the pub, and he was now a twenty-something responsible husband and father living 20 miles away, and the toaster's plug is now safely and securely wired up. Not very realistic, but hopefully giving you an idea.

Pat: *And is it something I could learn to do? Everything you've said so far makes so much sense to me that I'm seriously considering it. Is there a book I could read or could I download some scripts from the internet? Did you learn it from a correspondence course?*

Me: It takes a Home Study and a Practical Course to have any chance of gaining enough understanding of the theory and the practice to become a safe and effective practitioner. So it wouldn't be a good idea to put into a book the information that might allow anyone to assume they know how to treat people using this therapy. (...even someone as careful as you.)

That kind of detail needs to be given in an environment that monitors that learning process, assesses progress and supports an ongoing programme of continuous development and improvement. So this explanation is more to give an idea, paint a picture that gives an impression of how it works, rather than provide a step-by-step guide.

Pat: *So I'd need to go on a course, then?*

Me: If you want to start treating people, yes you would, but to understand more about it before you decide, I can fill in a few more details to help you along. It's a big decision to train or re-train as a therapist, and there are loads of different avenues to choose from. It's important to know whether it resonates with you and also whether you have the right skills, the right potential, the right motivation.

Pat: *There are bound to be easier ways to make a living, I guess. But so far, I'm interested and LCH has made it to my shortlist.*

Me: We start with an assumption that we're meant to be well and safe and happy - and with a belief that making that happen is the job of the subconscious mind. The subconscious part of our mind is our life-support system. If we're unhappy, unhealthy or accident-prone, then it's not that the subconscious mind is the enemy within. It's part of us, it IS us – so what is good for our subconscious mind should be good for us and vice versa. So we assume that it's doing what it's doing for some good reason and the best way to deal with that situation is to find that reason and put it under the microscope. We need to analyse it, find any hidden flaws or anything that's out of date, and assist in their correction or update.

If a computer program isn't working properly, we may know that there's a line of code that's invalid, or correct but in the wrong place, and even if we're right, that hasn't fixed it. We have to find that line of code, find out what's wrong with it or wrong with where it is. We have to make the appropriate amendment and then we have to re-run the program to see if that has fixed the problem.

LCH is that whole process – working with a human being who wants treatment rather than with a computer that's malfunctioning.

Pat: *I can only get on with computer analogies up to a point, and then my eyes glaze over and my mind flicks across to the 'what's for tea?' channel.*

Me: Ok, I get the hint – you'd like a more life-like example. We can study Judy. She has an addiction to chewing gum. She didn't have that addiction until 2 years ago. She doesn't like it because she thinks it looks so wrong in a forty-something professional woman and it's playing havoc with her digestion which is responding to that chewing motion by keeping her digestive system in a constant state of readiness for food that never arrives. So she doesn't want the addiction, she didn't choose it in the first place, she wants to stop the habit but can't. No amount of willpower can overcome those immense cravings that will only be satisfied by that tiny piece of sugar-coated rubber being constantly chewed.

Normally, she can choose what she eats and she is happy that she eats a healthy quantity and quality of food that leaves her feeling energised and satisfied. But over the past 2 years, she's found herself driven to buy and consume this gum each and every day – totally against her conscious wishes.

Pat: *So why is she doing it?*

Me: Her subconscious mind is in control. It's running a program that has now started to go wrong. She has a program in her, somewhere in her mind, her body, her brain, somewhere inside her is a program that is driving all her habits, taking care of all her routine tasks. We need to examine that program to find out why it's doing what it's doing.

Pat: *You've drifted back to your e-world. Come back into mine! Why did she create this habit? Why is this habit persisting in spite of her not wanting it?*

Me: Bear with me a bit longer. It won't be too painful, trust me.

This program is run by a computer. It relies on those instructions being correct and appropriate and in the right order. It normally doesn't, without some external guidance, re-examine those instructions once accepted and stored. It does a lot of testing before it stores them, but once stored, it uses them with confidence - it never questions them in any way.

So we need to re-examine those instructions...

We start with the symptom, the error message. We ask some questions...

and, based on the answers we get, that leads us to some more questions...

and, based on the answers we get, that leads us...

Pat: *Ok, I get the picture - but how do we know when to stop – how do we know when we've got there, when we've found that line of code that needs fixing?*

Me: You're right - unless the destination we're looking for is the airport or some huge out of town shopping centre, even when we get there, we could easily miss it.

There must be some kind of error in the line of code or in its position in the program. But it must also have been hidden in some way. If it had been obvious at the time, it would never have got past that rigorous testing. Something camouflaged it. In some way, it seemed plausible, believable, it made some kind of sense. Something, some detail, some other information enabled the flaw to sneak past all that testing and verifying and, like a virus, lie hidden and undetected in the depths of the computer until a particular set of data, a circumstance, some event or series of incidents caught its trip wire and let it loose to cause havoc.

We know we've got there when we find both the error itself and what caused it to get past the testing. Both ingredients are necessary. Without an error, then there's nothing to cause a problem. An obvious error wouldn't have been missed in the first place – it would have got corrected straight away.

Pat: *So then, is that it? Once we've found them both, once the patient knows why they have a problem, what caused it, does the symptom go away?*

Me: Well, no. Even if I know what's wrong with my computer and I know what needs to be done to fix it, it still needs fixing. If it involves some skills I don't have as a computer-user, my computer still won't be fixed.

And...

A techie, someone with all the right skills, can fix my computer without my understanding what was wrong or how it was fixed. So the techie starts with the symptom, we say what the computer is doing, or not doing, they do some investigation, they find the error – and they fix it.

My knowing what caused the problem doesn't fix it – it's neither a necessary nor a sufficient condition for the delivery of that happy outcome.

Pat: *I'm losing the plot. Bring it back to real life, please. I don't want a new job as a PC support technician.*

Me: Ok. That error is some incident or event that was experienced and interpreted in some kind of mistaken way. In most cases, we find that it was something that happened some time in the first 10 or 15 years of life, when we are learning about life and our place in it, so our interpretation of it could well have been suspect. It would have been based on a very small amount of experience and knowledge – and could well benefit from a more mature and reasoned re-interpretation.

In treatment, we (LCH therapists) shine a torch on that event and its interpretation, that line of code, and find what looks wrong to us. We point that out to the subconscious mind and assist it in the process of finding a better, a more up-to-date interpretation. On finding such an amendment or improvement, then we again help the subconscious mind along in the process of replacing the old interpretation with the new one – replacing the flawed line of code with the corrected one –and then prompting the subconscious, the computer, to re-run the program, to re-work the data.

Pat: *And is that it then?*

Me: Possibly. Once that processing is complete, if that misinterpretation had been the root cause, and the only cause, of the symptom, then the re-run program is likely to lead to the desired outcome. The program will then run perfectly and the conscious mind will be happy with the result. The symptom, condition or issue will begin to be corrected.

If that total success is not immediately visible, it could take a little time to evolve naturally, at a healthy, comfortable pace, but a small amount of improvement should be detectable and should grow. If there is no improvement, or if it's very slow and faltering, then there is likely to be another event or incident, another error in the program, another line or two of code to fix.

So we continue until that program does its test-run without a hitch, and our testing is rigorous and painstaking. We do all that is humanly possible with the current state of our knowledge and experience to get the best possible outcome, the most benefit for the longest period of time – always aiming for 'happily ever after' and getting some remarkable feedback that sometimes includes expressions like 'life-changing'.

Pat: *All those computer references have caused my eyes to glaze over. They've left me with more questions than answers.*

Me: No worries – we can just as easily look at it from a different angle. We ask some questions. We want to know why the symptom or condition or issue has developed or been created and why something unwanted, uncomfortable, unhealthy, inconvenient has not been resolved.

Pat: *Yes but if it's a physical symptom like a pain, something visible like a rash, something functional like a breathing difficulty, then it could have been caused by some outside agent like an injury, a virus, an allergen.*

Me: That's true but we have a wonderful healing, balancing, correcting mechanism within us that, given time and the right environment, in the huge majority of cases, manages to fix such externally-generated undesirables even before most of them ever reach our conscious awareness.

Pat: *So if the condition doesn't improve over time, there must be a reason?*

Me: That's what I believe.

Pat: *And why do you believe that? I find your examples usually help me get it more easily.*

Me: Ok. So, for example...

Most people in many parts of the world walk around in shoes most of the time, and walk around bare-footed on occasions. The skin on the soles of our feet is just strong enough to cope with those kinds of demands. For the people in the habit of walking around without footwear most of the day, then the skin is much tougher, much stronger, so that the contact with the ground doesn't cause discomfort or damage.

Pat: *Ok so far.*

Me: And if we were to move from one environment or custom to the other then, given time, our feet would adapt.

Pat: *Yes I agree - given time and depending on our age. We adapt more quickly when we are younger.*

Me: If we take up guitar-playing, as I did many years ago, especially the metal-stringed variety, then at first, we would only be able to practice for a short

46

time each day before pain in the finger ends set in. Pressing on those strings is very uncomfortable for the novice. Gradually, the pain reduces and the student is able to play for longer periods each day. An examination of those finger-ends shows a kind of hard skin developing just like that on the soles of the feet of the barefoot walker. This causes the nerve endings to be a little further away, to be insulated by that harder skin, from those narrow and unyielding metal edges.

Pat: *So is the subconscious protecting the tissue by making it tougher, and making it less painful so the student can practice more?*

Me: Yes and should the student give up on the daily practice, again from my own experience, then steadily, day by day, that hard skin begins to reduce, to shrink, to get thinner, until it returns to its pre-guitar level.

So if we make different demands of our bodies, if we put ourselves in new surroundings that are warmer or cooler, harsher or milder, noisier or quieter, then our bodies adapt, over time, to cope as well as is humanly possible with the environment. If we go to a new country, or even a new planet, we have no immunity to the bacteria, infections, viruses that live there, so we may become very ill. If that illness doesn't kill us, we become tougher and gain the immunity to those previously unfamiliar bugs.

And in a population of millions, if a virus were so infectious that many caught it, then we'd still have loads of people who stayed well enough to look after the sick and keep the whole show on the road. Those hardy folk have immune systems so powerful and adaptable, so quick to learn, that even the most virulent and least familiar germs would be zapped before they had a chance of getting a foot in the door.

So if we're always catching colds whenever there's one going around, or if we're always the first to catch pneumonia and yet we're as tough as old boots when it comes to walking on the hills in all weathers, love the wind and the rain and all that the sky can throw at us, then the chances are that there's some reason for our particular Achilles' heel.

Pat: *Ok I'm still with you on your theory that there has to be a reason if we get ill and don't, in time, recover – but again, what has that got to do with your patients? They come to you for hypnotherapy, and there's a limited range of conditions that people associate with that kind of treatment.*

Me: You're right, and in the same way, if we aren't adapting to our circumstances and if common sense and willpower fail to sort things out for us, if we aren't getting better at what we practice, there has to be something that explains it.

If we panic over the slightest hint of having to speak in public, even to ask for a coffee in a cafe, if we run a mile from that tiny money-spider that others happily pick up and carry outside, if we lie in bed each night, tired, exhausted, but wide awake and alert while the rest of the family snore away gently around us, if that packet of biscuits in the cupboard is calling to us when we know we've just had a good and nutritious meal and no-one else could face another mouthful – whatever is our personal psychological tug-of-war – then there must be something that explains it.

Pat: *Could it just be a coincidence, just random, like the colour of our eyes?*

Me: Yes it could, but I'd always want to know why it started when it did. If we weren't born with it, then something must have triggered it off. And if you pull the trigger and there's no bullet in the gun, then all you get is a little click. So something must have put the bullet in the gun in the first place for that trigger-pulling to have caused such a long-lasting after-effect.

In the 20+ years of my career as a computer programmer, I never once found an error that occurred for no reason. I always eventually found the line of code, the logic error, the data inconsistency that made it all make sense. In the early days, I needed a lot of help, but gradually managed with less and less assistance, and however big and complex a program, it is only a collection of lines of code processing some input from some files or from some keystrokes or mouse-clicks.

Pat: *You're off on your computer stuff again!*

Me: I know, but hopefully it's the Reader's Digest or Twitter version – short and sweet and low on techno-babble.

Pat: *Ok, I'll give you that – just don't get carried away.*

Me: Our bodies are far more complex and self-balancing than any computer outside of science-fiction, so my own personal belief is that nothing ever 'just happens'. It's just that we haven't found all the causes yet. But we have found a lot of them and we're getting better at it all the time.

Pat: *And how do we find the cause?*

Me: A good place to start is to ask some questions. We need to ask 'Why?' – but it's not that easy. We need to find the right questions - and we need to find the right 'person' to ask those questions of – and we need to set up a line of communication with that 'person' – and we need to establish a common language.

Pat: *Sounds pretty complicated.*

Me: Yes but it's all included in that comprehensive training program. This is just to give you an idea, not to get you ready to treat patients.

Pat: *Ok. I think I'll send off for a prospectus. I need to hear some of this from the people who do the teaching. Carry on.*

Me: We have to start somewhere, so how about first looking at the questions - what we want to know and what we know already. We know the symptom or condition or issue or whatever we want to call it. We know what the patient or client wants fixing. And if we simply ask the patient why they have that symptom, then they might be able to tell us.

Pat: *Example please....*

Me: Simon has insomnia and he believes it's because
he has money worries. His company is on the
rocks and he wakes up in the night with his mind
whizzing round and chattering away about all
the things that are going wrong and no solutions
spring to mind – it's all doom and gloom. He
knows that the lack of sleep and resulting daytime
exhaustion are making it even harder for him to
turn his business around - so he wants me to fix it,
to press that switch that makes him revert to the
kind of sleep pattern he had as a student when he
could fall asleep at a party with music so loud the
neighbours have complained.

Pat: *Well you can't fix the recession from your
consulting room, can you?*

Me: No but when I ask a few more questions, it
emerges that he can worry for England. If the
profits are rolling in, he'll worry about his taxes.
If his order books are full, he'll fear a change in
fashion that will take his customers away. If his
wife goes out and buys some new clothes, he's
convinced it's to impress some secret lover.

Pat: *And if someone were to discuss it with him,
suggest other explanations for his life experiences,
offer rational arguments for how counter-
productive are his anxieties and pessimism, he
might easily agree.*

Me: Yes and he's probably told himself the same and
heard it from any friends and family in whom he's
confided. But maybe he needed to hear it from
someone neutral, someone with qualifications and

experience in such matters - a professional, a counsellor, a talking therapy of some kind such as Cognitive Behavioural Therapy.

Pat: *I understand that many of these types of therapy deliver remarkable results. Is that more likely to be what he needs?*

Me: Maybe - but in some cases they don't work. Or they work for a while but then, after treatment has been concluded, old habits can begin to return and people can slip back into their old ways.

Pat: *So if that happens, then is there likely to be another layer?*

Me: Yes, maybe it goes deeper. Maybe it's not subject to rational thought or maybe it's not manageable by will-power – or maybe managing it takes a huge amount of time and energy that could be better spent on working and playing.

Pat: *So if CBT or counselling or psychotherapy work for some people, then they don't need your LCH – is that what you're saying?*

Me: From my own personal clinical viewpoint, I'm happy to treat people from 2 sets of circumstances – those who have tried everything else and nothing has worked for them – and those who understand the theory of LCH and, like me, see its logic and simplicity as reassuring and compelling.

If some other treatment works, if the symptom never returns or gets replaced by another one (but it isn't always obvious if a symptom is a replacement) then that is fantastic. But some treatments require a patient to re-open old wounds, to dig around and find that piece of hidden shrapnel, to cry and shout and let off steam – and that wouldn't be my choice if there was another way.

Pat: *Hmmm... me neither.*

Me: So that's another reason to give LCH a try. It involves the mental equivalent of handing your car keys to the mechanic and enjoying a cappuccino in a riverside cafe until that call comes through on your mobile to say your car is serviced and fixed and ready for you to drive away. There's just the little matter of the bill to pay.

Pat: *I like the sound of that.*

Me: So we need to find the right questions and ask those questions of the right 'person'.

Pat: *We're back to the subconscious again, right?*

Me: Yes, because if not, if it just took some common sense and maybe someone to talk it over with, then he, or at least, his friends and family, would have already resolved it.

Pat: *So you ask the subconscious mind some questions?*

Me: Yes - and it takes a few steps to get there. Think about the symptom or condition as being the start of a treasure hunt. Think about the cause of that symptom as being the treasure itself. In a treasure hunt, we all set off with the same initial clue – the symptom – in our example, insomnia. We know there has to be a reason why it exists because, like the extra layer of skin on the fingers of the ex-guitar-player, if it's no longer required, it gradually disappears.

Pat: *So we ask why it's needed?*

Me: Yes but we can't just ask our patient. He doesn't know the full story because if he did, he wouldn't now be needing treatment. He doesn't want it, and as far as he's aware, he doesn't need it, and nothing he has been able to think of up to now has fully resolved it for him. He wants a good night's sleep and a refreshed and alert start to his day.

His thoughts and memories might make some kind of sense of this condition, but so far, nothing has taken it away. That thinking, deciding, analyzing, choosing, conscious part of his mind has done all it can and drawn a blank.

Pat: *So we have to ask the other part of his mind, the subconscious part – but how can we do that?*

Me: It's a bit like relationship counselling. We need to get the talkative or bossy one in a couple (the conscious mind) to keep quiet and we need to help the quiet or shy and nervous one (the subconscious mind) to speak out when they've never been asked before and they don't know if they want to and they imagine their voice will be shaky and what they say will be laughed at or shouted down.

Pat: *Takes a bit of time, then?*

Me: Yes it takes a session or two to build up. It takes a bit of reassurance that the quiet voice will have a supportive and understanding audience–and it takes a bit of persuasion to get the chatty one to go off and get a coffee or walk the dog - and it takes a bit of explanation that the couple will get on a lot better afterwards.

Pat: *And how do you do that?*

Me: We ask the chatty one to take a relaxing break that leaves them feeling like they can't be bothered to butt in, haven't followed the proceedings so wouldn't know what to say, have lost the drift of the conversation and anyway, this daydream is much more interesting. Imagine a teenager watching TV and being asked loads of questions about how school went that day. They keep their eyes glued to the screen and mutter yes/no or lift their shoulders in a shrug of 'whatever'. That's the hypnosis part. We use a hypnotic induction to help our patients reach the 'can't be bothered' state that most will recognise from Sunday morning. "I'll get out of bed – in a while..."

Pat: *So you get information from the subconscious mind that way – and I'm guessing the questions in my mind, "how on earth...?" would be answered by the formal training.*

Me: That's right - but let's stick to the investigation process for now. Once we get the answer that helps us complete the first stage of that treasure hunt, then wherever that is, it gives us the beginnings of an idea of what to ask in order to set off on the second stage. We have a bit of structure to go on.

Pat: *Help!!!*

Me: We're on a journey, starting out with the route-planning map and setting off from the motorway services. There are huge blue signs telling us which direction to go for all the major destinations. We can stay on the motorway network for miles before an answer takes us onto an A-road, where it becomes slightly more challenging – there are loads more of them and they go all over, but there are still clear signposts to guide us. Again, we can go many miles on A-roads until an answer takes us to a B-road.

Once on the B-road, we could find ourselves on an unmarked road in the countryside or a street, avenue or crescent in the middle of a huge residential estate. In the countryside, we might need to get out of the car and start walking along a path, but that might peter out and leave us with no option but to scramble through the heather and brambles until we find that particular pebble that our patient tripped over back in 1974.

Pat: *That was that incident?*

Me: Yes - in treatment, we can reach our destination so easily because it was in the reception of a motel at the next motorway service station, or it was in the kitchen of the pub at the junction of the A123 and the B4567, but equally, it could take a lot more searching because it was in a cardboard box in the cupboard under the stairs behind the vacuum-cleaner and the step-ladder in 432 Misplacement Avenue, Warningtown-on-Sea - we have no idea. We just have to keep asking questions and following directions.

Pat: *So it's quite complex then? If I'm going to train in LCH, I need to like a challenge, is that right?*

Me: Yes – exactly right. One reason for that detailed and multi-faceted training course is that, without it, it's so easy to go wrong. Using that same analogy that finding the error is like following directions to find a geographical location...

I need to go from A to G and have some step by step directions: -

Start at A

To get to B - take first left

To get to C - at next traffic lights, go straight on

To get to D – take second right

To get to E - at next roundabout, turn right

To get to F – take second left

To reach destination of G – continue straight on for 100 yards and see your destination directly opposite a large and famous retail outlet – you can't miss it

Ok let's give it a go...

Start at A

To get to B - take first left – got that ok

To get to C - at next traffic lights, go straight on – ok got that

To get to D – take second right – ok

To get to E - at next roundabout, turn right – yep that's fine too

To get to F – take second left – ok

To reach destination of G – continue straight on for 100 yards and see your destination directly opposite a large and famous retail outlet – you can't miss it – errrr… no sign of that big shop – I found myself down some unlit road to nowhere - and knowing that my destination was in the city centre, had to go back and ask for some more help.

It emerged that I'd taken the second right after the first a set of **traffic lights** rather than noting the earlier set of **pedestrian lights** and taking the second right after those. But both **could** be referred to as traffic lights as they both look similar and both control the traffic. So having learnt that I need to check which kind of traffic lights, I started out from the beginning and got a bit further….

Start at A

To get to B - take first left – got that ok

To get to C - at next **pedestrian crossing traffic lights,** go straight on – ok got that

To get to D – take second right – ok

To get to E - at next roundabout, turn right – yep that's fine too

To get to F – take second left – ok

To reach destination of G – continue straight on for 100 yards and see your destination directly opposite a large and famous retail outlet – you can't miss it – errrr...still no sign of that big shop – I found myself in an industrial estate with no shops in sight, so had to go back and ask for some more help.

Turn right at the roundabout - there were 5 roads into that roundabout, and that gave 2 possible right turns. I took the first of those two - not seeing the second which was a small unmarked road. The road I took was an A-road – easy to spot, an obvious choice, but I didn't check out if that was the one.

(Checking the information in more detail, more thoroughly). Ok is this the only right turn? No.

Ok is the right turn that I want an A-road? No.

Ok so do I want the minor unmarked road? Yes.

Second left OK

100 yards further on there's this huge brightly lit retail giant and I'm smiling to myself as I see my destination straight opposite – I couldn't miss it.

Pat: *And back to your patients – how is that relevant to LCH? What's the connection?*

Me: Pedestrian lights and Traffic lights look the same and have a similar function but if I'm seeing them as the same thing and my patient's subconscious mind is seeing them as 2 different things, or vice versa, I'll set off down the wrong path.

I wasn't counting the pedestrian lights and my patient's subconscious was.

Roundabouts can have any number of exits. I had assumed 4. I had also only looked for the major roads.

Main lessons: -

1. It doesn't matter how I define something – it's how my patient's subconscious mind defines it that matters.

2. Just like in a court of law, the subconscious mind can only answer the questions I've asked. To prevent a miscarriage of justice, I need to give my witness the opportunity to provide **all** relevant information.

Pat: *I'm getting the idea, a bit, but can you make it more realistic?*

Me: No, I'm continuing to be vague so as not to provide a 'teach yourself LCH' book, I'm not going to spell out what kind of 'real-life' example this could relate to in treatment. It's just to create an image, so like that singing, humming, chirpy Australian artist so often says, "Can you tell what it is yet?"

Pat: *Doh!*

Me: And that complexity, that potential for taking wrong turnings, is why it takes such a detailed and varied training program and a therapist with an inquisitive nature and an attention to detail and a tenacity to keep going even when the map can't help and we need other equipment like a compass, some stars and a trust that we can pitch our tent for the night and pick up the trail when the light returns the next day.

Pat: *So if I prefer to spend my working hours following a set of detailed instructions designed and written up by someone else and having someone to refer to as soon as something even slightly out of the ordinary comes along - and if I prefer to hand it over to someone else to fix rather than even begin to try to work it out for myself, then maybe this isn't for me?*

Me: Maybe – but unless you've had a personality transplant since our student days, I'm not expecting that any of that refers to you. You'd need to have a mind that likes a challenge about subjects that are real, affecting real people, with a real chance of making a real difference.

Pat: *No worries – the prospectus request is in the post. Carry on slapping paint on canvas with that 3 inch emulsion brush. It's starting to look like a kangaroo.*

Me: Ok. Each leg of the treasure hunt can be likened to the point at which you leave that class of road. There has been some confirmation that that particular stage has been reached and that we have a direction arrow to help us set off for the next one.

Pat: *And how do we know when we've got there?*

Me: When we finally reach the treasure, we and our patient may have a Eureka moment, or it may be that it takes a few days or weeks for the light to come on. The subconscious mind can cause a sense of relief, a lightening of an accustomed load, a feeling of closure – or it can also be that nothing at all is experienced by the patient but the therapist gets a quiet word from the treasure-hunt organiser – 'it's ok, you can go home now, you've cracked it and your prize will arrive in the post in the next 28 days'.

The patient goes home with your words of reassurance – the roots of those weeds, or at least some of them, have been dug up, so let's leave it a few weeks to settle and see how the garden looks after that. Even then, when the patient returns, maybe no smiles of relief, no words of thanks, they just turn up, sit down and wait for you to work some more magic on them. You ask for some feedback. 'How has your symptom been? Any changes?'

And if all the roots had been found and the garden had been cleared of that weed, then it can be as noticeable as a clean and tidy house.

Pat: *Yes I get that one. My lot only notice when it's dirty and things are out of place and they can't find things. Otherwise they've no idea what I've been doing all day while they were out at the park with a football.*

Me: Gradually it emerges that that symptom that had been a constant unwelcome companion several times a day for many years had reduced in the last few weeks to daily, then every few days and they can't actually remember the last time....

On the whole, after a further check for any stray and hidden roots, that's the time to smile and predict that they aren't likely to need you again because things look like they are proceeding nicely. And if they do, then a return for the disposal of any stray or loose ends might just be needed and they know where to find you.

If the problem is big,
then is the cause big too?

Now it's time for Chris to turn up and Pat has had to go back to unrewarding housework and ungrateful lodgers. And you might want to watch out for when you get Pat and Chris in the same room at the same time. Hmmm...

Pat and Chris are always chatting to each other, and recently, the subject has often had some connection to LCH. Chris has a fear of driving that has only developed over the past couple of years, and before that, was confident and competent in the driving seat.

Chris: *Pat was suggesting that you might be able to help me with my fear of driving. It's getting worse all the time, and last week, I got a full-blown panic attack at the wheel and only just managed to pull over to the side. My partner was with me and had to take over for the rest of the journey. It was horrible and I haven't driven since. My heart was pounding, I felt sick, I couldn't focus properly and I thought I was going to faint.*

  Me: Pat's right, I might be able to help.

Chris: Pat also says that LCH works by finding and resolving the underlying cause.

Me: Again, that's right.

Chris: Well I know why I've got it. I was a passenger in a bus a few years ago, and we skidded on some ice and nearly ended up in the ditch. I've been a bit nervous ever since and it's been getting steadily worse. That near-miss is what caused it. I just need some help to get over it.

Me: I agree that your scary incident on the bus has something to do with it, but I disagree that that was the cause.

Chris: How can you be so sure?

Me: How many other passengers were there on the bus with you?

Chris: About 30 or so.

Me: Were any of them actually with you, or were any of them people that you know?

Chris: Yes, I can remember at least 2.

Me: And do you know if they now have a fear of driving?

Chris: No I don't think they do.

Me: And would you imagine that all of those others, the ones you didn't know, would you imagine that all or even most of those also now have a fear of driving? Is a fear of driving that common?

Chris: *No I don't suppose that's likely.*

Me: So there must be more to it, then. There must be something that explains why you reacted in the way that you did and most other passengers on that same journey didn't. And this time I can give you a real-life example. - something that actually happened to me. This one isn't fiction.

A few years ago, I was driving down the motorway on my way to a conference and was at a point where the motorway divided into 2 roads and as I wanted the right hand road, I manoeuvred over to the third lane of five. That was to become the left hand lane of the right hand road, but the two lanes to the left of me were open to traffic wanting the left hand road, traffic that was potentially travelling faster than I was.

Chris: *Ok, I think I can picture it.*

Me: At that point, I lost all power! The accelerator was right down to the floor but nothing was coming through. I was losing momentum rapidly.

Chris: *That must have been terrifying!*

Me: I didn't have time to be terrified at that point. That hit me a bit later on. I realised I had to act quickly. I put the hazard lights on to warn the surrounding traffic that they might need to get out of my way, quickly glanced around but didn't see anything close to me, so I started to coast across two lanes and onto the hard shoulder. I got there safely and spent the first

few minutes saying thank you to whoever or
whatever had been looking after me.

I got out of the car and sat on the grass
embankment and watched those two lanes that
I had just coasted across. There wasn't another
gap in the traffic like the one that had saved me
in the whole of the time I sat waiting for the
recovery man.

Chris: *I couldn't have got back in the car after that.
That was much worse than that skidding bus.
Did you have to have treatment?*

Me: I've had treatment, but I didn't need any for
that experience. The recovery man needed all
his patience and reassurance to get me back in
the car to continue my journey. I was shaken
and very scared, and made sure I stayed in the
left hand lane as much as possible, making sure
there was nothing between me and the hard
shoulder.

I had the car thoroughly checked when I got
back. They found and corrected the fault and
I took a bit of time building up my confidence
once again. Eventually, I ventured onto the
motorway again, and found myself on that
same 5-lane section, again in the middle lane.

I was very nervous.

Chris: *I'm not surprised.*

Me: No, it's not surprising that a recent ordeal, such
a dramatic near-miss, would affect anyone the

first time they found themselves in similar circumstances, but I was ok – nothing happened. The next time I was in the same place, I was still nervous, but not quite so much. The fact that I had been fine the next time had reduced the fear and anticipation.

And after a few trips, over a few weeks, I stopped reacting to that stretch of road. I had just about forgotten it in a few months.

Chris: *So are you saying that that is the normal reaction – to steadily get over it?*

Me: I don't know what is normal, but it seems to make sense to me that subsequent safe journeys should reduce rather than increase that fear. What do you think?

Chris: *Yes I suppose so. I've had other things happen to me and got over them like you did. So why am I acting differently with driving? Do you think there's something that caused me to react that way – something that made me react differently from all those other passengers? Is that what you mean by the underlying cause?*

Me: Yes, something like that.

Chris: *Well then, I'm not sure if I want to go there. That panic attack was so severe and I felt so bad that the underlying cause is likely to be something huge – isn't that right? I wouldn't be suffering that much over something small, would I?*

And...

Why can't you treat the symptom directly and ignore the cause? After all, it's in the past, so how can it still be causing a problem? Why do I have to spend time on revisiting the past when all I really need to do is deal with my problems here and now?

Me: Most of my patients only take the time and trouble to look for help, only consider spending money on some therapy, when they've got to the end of their tether, when their condition is severe and deeply life-affecting. Many initially think the way you do right now – and it's quite understandable to make that assumption - that a huge problem is likely to have had an equally huge cause.

People worry if there's some skeleton in their cupboard, some trauma hidden deep, well away from their memory. They feel anxious that they might recall some secret event that happened when they were very young - something so awful that the subconscious mind has hidden it away to protect them from the pain, something they would be most unwilling to re-visit.

So I can explain it to you in the same kind of way I use for my patients. I use a lot of analogies, and I use one which is a real-life example of a big problem with a tiny cause.

Chris: *Well I can't think of any, so go on, surprise me.*

Me: Imagine a house which has a water-pipe with a tiny crack in it. The crack is in a section of pipe that is under the floor-boards, and it is so tiny that it only allows a drop of water to escape every day or so. To the untrained eye, the crack is too small to be seen. Left to release that tiny amount of water for 20 years or more, you would end up with a house with rotting floorboards, wet plaster, wallpaper falling off, and a constant all-pervading smell of damp. That's a pretty big problem from a cause so tiny that it's invisible to everyone but the plumber.

Chris: Hmmm... ok. That sounds plausible.

Me: And in this case, we could directly treat the symptom without also fixing the underlying cause. We could bring in the de-humidifiers and replace the plaster and the floorboards, and we could redecorate throughout, but that will only buy a little relief before it all sets in again. Once the cause, that tiny crack in the pipe, is fixed, then we can happily do all that restorative work and it's likely to stay good for a very long time.

Chris: Ok – Pat said you had an answer for everything. But what makes you so confident that that's likely to be the case for your patients?

Me: It just seems logical to me, and it's been borne out by years of clinical practice. Going on with the cracked pipe analogy, the reason it persists for so long is BECAUSE it's so tiny – it's so hard to find. If the pipe were to crack open completely and water were to gush out, we would have no trouble finding the source of all that water, and we'd be extremely unlikely to ignore it and leave it uncorrected. Something big and dramatic is more likely to get lots of attention very early on.

We might ignore a tiny niggling irritation in the shoulder, and we might get so used to it that we no longer notice it, or we might discover that if we limit our movement, there's no pain, and then we might forget that we adjusted our posture in the name of comfort and carry on happily for years without getting any help - but the pain of a heart attack will not be ignored, and whatever we do, it won't go away until we get the appropriate medical intervention.

So a big problem can easily have a tiny cause, and a big cause is unlikely to lead to a problem because it will receive the appropriate care and attention straight away and not be left under the floorboards to create a puzzling damp patch and a musty smell.

Chris: *Is that a bit like when you get some grit in your shoe or in your eye, or when you develop a hole in a tooth or filling? They seem much bigger than they really are.*

Me: Yes, grit in my shoe is a good example. Let's pursue that one and see where it takes us.

I know it's there because it hurts when I walk, but when I take off my shoe, check my shoe and my sock, I can't find the culprit. I'm in a hurry, got a train to catch, no time to keep searching, so I put the shoe back on and hope that the grit has been dislodged and fallen out. But no, it must still be there because it still hurts. There's a sharp, stabbing pain in my heel.

I rush around for the rest of the day, no time to stop and search properly. But because it hurts so much and I need to do so much walking, I find that I can get by and that it hurts less if I don't put so much weight on that heel. By the end of the day, I'm automatically walking with my heel slightly raised. It's something we all do automatically. We adjust to reduce or remove pain if at all possible.

The next day, it happens again. I try again to find that piece of grit. It must be there because if I put my weight fully down on that heel, the pain is just as severe, just as sharp. And I'm even busier today but it's ok, I know what to do. I walk with the heel slightly raised, and that's becoming a bit easier with practice.

The third day, I'm only vaguely aware of it. I'm automatically adopting that unusual gait, and I'm more aware now of a pain in my knee. I have no time to think of that piece of grit because my knee is starting to grumble and ache and demand my attention. This time I have to go to the pharmacists and buy a support bandage. That gives it some support and eases the pain.

And the days turn into weeks. I've forgotten the piece of grit and the pain in the heel, and each time I try to do without my bandage, the pain returns. But the bandage prevents me from bending my knee as much as I need to in order to walk comfortably and naturally on the flat, and in order to walk up and down stairs I need to always keep that one leg fairly straight.

To keep the leg straight but still manage to travel effectively from A to B, I need to lean away from that strapped up knee and swing my hip a little to propel the affected leg forwards. Once my hip gets used to that, the pain recedes.

I reach a state where all of this becomes automatic. I lift my heel, I wear my bandage, I keep that leg fairly straight and swing my hip forwards a little when I walk. I'm sure you can see the pattern evolving. Each problem is fixed by an adjustment in some other part of the body.

This continues upwards, moving through back-pain, shoulder-ache and eventually, a stiff and immobile neck. At that point, it has nowhere else to go. Nothing else can adjust to ease the discomfort or provide that necessary mobility.

If this were you, what would you be doing now? You suggested that there's no need to look into the past, just treat the present symptom, so what would you do in that case.

Chris: *I guess I'd go for treatment for my neck pain.*

Me: But in this case, a direct treatment for the neck, its pain and stiffness, is not going to be successful, because this particular neck pain was caused by a tiny piece of grit.

Chris: *Yes I can see it in that case.*

Me: Once that grit is found and removed, then the heel can learn to relax and take the body weight again, without pain. Once the heel is resting in the shoe as before, the knee is no longer pulled out of alignment, so I find I can take off the bandage eventually without the pain returning. Without the bandage and without the pain, the knee can move more and I can bend and flex the knee freely again. With the knee moving now in the way it was meant to, I no longer need to swing my hip to move that leg forward. And with all of those adjustments corrected again, the back, shoulder and neck begin to return to the comfort and degree of movement I'd enjoyed before.

So in this case, the only fully effective way of resolving the symptom in the long term, dare I say permanently, and to prevent it getting replaced by yet another symptom each time, is to find and undo the original error – put the grit back where it belongs – outside.

Chris: *Yes I agree with that, but what makes you so sure it would be as small as a tiny piece of grit?*

Me: If that had been a bigger piece of grit, I wouldn't have struggled to find it. My fingers would have detected it and removed it easily on the first attempt. This whole sorry saga would have never started. And if, rather than a fair-sized piece of grit, it had been a pebble, or a stone, or a boulder, it would have never made it into my shoe in the first place. So again, the smaller the problem, the more it is able to hide and lead to puzzling symptoms months or years later.

Chris: *Ok, I agree it could be like that, but that was just one convenient example – one that fitted your theory. Surely it's just as likely to be something completely different?*

Me: I agree that it's just one example, so here's another one - an example of when there is little chance of achieving long-term relief by treating symptoms without resolving what caused them in the first place. Consider the case of someone with heart disease. The best that medical science can offer, the triple by-pass or even a transplant, the arteries fully cleared of plaque, will only provide temporary relief if the lifestyle pattern that created that unhealthy heart and circulation isn't corrected as well. If the diet and exercise pattern is left unchanged, if the emotional response to stress remains at red-alert, it will re-line those arteries and wear out that new and healthy heart before too long.

Chris: *A bit like all that work on the house with the cracked pipe still leaking?*

Me: Yes, it's very similar. We all know about healthy living and the effects of our diet and exercise patterns on our health, particularly on the heart and circulation, and we can try to do all the right things but some of us find ourselves unable to make the changes and keep them.

And as an ex-computer programmer, I hold a belief that nothing ever goes wrong without a reason. And yes, once the reason is corrected, we might have to do some work to fix the after-effects of that original cause, but I would never want to fix the after-effects until I had made as sure as I possibly could that the cause, the causes, the whole of the error was completely understood and the code itself was fully fixed, and that a thorough series of tests had been successfully completed.

Would you?

Chris: *No, I suppose not. But I'm not that used to computers, so if you're going to use them to explain something, you'll have to make it very simple and not technical.*

Me: Ok. I'll try.

Chris: *And what if I've got some deeply disturbing memories in that hidden part of my mind. I've read that treatment can unearth these and leave the patient traumatised. Do you think I might have something hidden like that?*

Me: There could well be all sorts of information that's long-forgotten, but for it to have been forgotten, then it's most likely to be because it was small and trivial.

And alternatively, if there were some childhood incident which would serve no good purpose to either the conscious or the subconscious mind to be reviewed or re-visited, then the subconscious mind would be doing its job by leaving it alone, letting that particular sleeping dog lie.

And LCH therapists do the same. If there's no purpose to be served, no gain to be had from finding and reviewing such a long-forgotten experience, then LCH treatment will, by its rigorous method, take the quickest route past such events to the information that is likely to have the best effect on reaching the desired outcome.

Chris: *And what about someone who had an extremely unhappy childhood, the kind you read about in the papers?*

Me: If someone is having nightmares about a trauma they lived through, then the sufferer needs help, support and understanding.

As far as I understand it, and I'm not trained or qualified in that type of therapy, for someone who has lived through any kind of trauma, the best chance they have of moving on quickly from disturbing memories and flashbacks is to work with someone trained in that field as soon as possible after the trauma. If that kind of help isn't received until much later in life, then the response might be slower, they might need more support, but there would still be an improvement, a lessening of the after-effects and a steady return towards a happier and more peaceful future.

And after that kind of support and therapy, they might then be able to say to themselves, "I know it happened. I know how much I suffered. But that's years ago and I've worked through it now. I've resolved it all and come to terms with it all now. I'm determined not to let it affect my life any longer. I'm not going to continue suffering because of it. I'm ready to move on now."

Chris: *Yes I'm sure people would like to say that, but how many of them can?*

Me: I don't know, but I believe there are some! I've heard and read of many people who have survived and thrived in spite of childhood pain and suffering, so if that suffering were the cause, then no one would survive it and go on to have a happy, healthy life. Think about my motorway experience. I steadily recovered from it. Like an infection, cut or a burn getting better, like a sprained ankle getting stronger, the subconscious mind is designed to heal psychological wounds as well as physical ones. That's what it's designed to do and that's what, in most cases, it succeeds in doing.

Chris: *Yes, you recovered from something that sounds more severe than my bus skidding, so I agree there must be some reason why my reaction was more severe and long lasting than yours. But I'm talking about something far more serious than that.*

Me: Yes I know, and I still believe that there are people who have recovered from experiences that I couldn't even begin to imagine or describe.

Chris: *I've read of such heroes too, but aren't they the exception that proves the rule?*

Me: I've never understood that expression, and no, I disagree. If something is the cause, is necessary and sufficient to predict a specific outcome, then an exception such as someone surviving and thriving after a traumatic childhood means that such a childhood doesn't necessarily lead to suffering as an adult. There has to be something that explains why some people suffer later on in life and others don't.

Such a childhood could easily trigger a symptom, but pulling the trigger of a gun that has no bullet in it is unlikely to have any lasting negative results. I believe that those who suffer as adults have a bullet in their gun. And if they had seen the bullet being placed in the gun, they, or others taking care of them, would have removed the bullet and disposed of it. They, or their adult carers, guardians, teachers, someone would have made sure that they weren't left with a loaded gun lying around just waiting to be accidentally triggered.

Chris: *I'm not sure. Can you relate it to real life for me?*

Me: The incident that loaded the gun, the event that set up that situation where a trauma would have lasting and puzzling after-effects, must have had some quality that camouflaged it in some way. There must have been something about it that made it seem sensible and appropriate. And you can only hide a small error. If it was big, then it would have had loads of attention – it couldn't have slipped by unnoticed.

Chris: *Ok but there must be loads of types of symptoms that LCH can't fix.*

Me: Of course there are. If I witnessed a horrific road accident and had nightmares for months afterwards, then I would need help and support to recover from that ordeal. If I was injured in that crash, I would need the best that our health system can offer to heal those wounds and to recuperate, but I wouldn't be looking to solve some mystery, I wouldn't be wondering why I was in pain, physical or psychological or both. I would know why and there is plenty of expertise around to deal with my suffering and aid my recovery.

Chris: *So how can you tell if LCH is the right therapy for someone?*

Me: I usually rely on finding something puzzling, something that seems to make no sense to me. If I suffer earache for months or even years, and if no medical test has ever detected any reason for that pain, then there's something puzzling going on. I would want to know why and would expect that LCH would be likely to help resolve it.

As soon as I find myself puzzled, as soon as I ask myself "why?" - that's when I think about LCH, expecting to find that the cause was as small and easily missable as that tiny crack in the water pipe or that irritating piece of grit.

Chris: *So my fear of driving. I agree with you now, it's puzzling that I haven't got over the bus skidding, so do you think you could help me with that?*

Me: Probably.

Best friend

Chris: *Pat has told me a bit about the subconscious being like a personal assistant, but what would make a personal assistant cause me to panic rather than get over my scary journey?*

Me: The personal assistant is just one way of describing the subconscious. I use various different descriptions that seem to illustrate the way the subconscious works in various different circumstances.

Chris: *Ok so what would explain that escalating response?*

Me: Imagine the subconscious mind as a best friend and we'll see if that gives us some clues.

My friend Amy is always there for me, would do anything for me. She's always on my side, sticking up for me, putting herself out to help me if I ask, and even when I don't, seems to know instinctively what I want or need and just arranges it all for me. But mysteriously, from time to time, she says or does something that upsets me, hurts me, causes me some inconvenience or worse, and I wonder why.

I don't think angry thoughts about her. I'm not tempted to say something sharp and cutting to her. I don't even feel frustrated or irritated. I'm simply puzzled. What had gone wrong? Was there some misunderstanding? Had she misunderstood – or had I? Was there something she, or I, didn't know about, something that explained this rare and out-of-character behaviour?

It would make sense to find out before asking for a change in her behaviour. Maybe she was doing the right thing. Maybe it was for my own good.

Chris: I'm beginning to get the idea, but an example would probably help it along.

Me: Last year, one lovely summer's afternoon, Amy and I were sitting in the garden together, chatting away happily when a ladybird landed on the arm of my garden recliner. I noticed it and, as many people do, I put my finger in front of it, in its path, for it to walk over. It's something that is pleasant, something so small and pretty, so tiny that you can't actually feel its presence as it walks over your finger.

Chris: Yes I do that too.

Me: Imagine how surprised and concerned I was when Amy told me to get my hand away, and seemed quite agitated. She was beside herself. She told me I mustn't let that insect touch me. I tried to reassure her, not sure what danger she believed I was in, or why. It was just a harmless ladybird.

But she wouldn't be pacified and as the insect got nearer, she jumped up and knocked my hand off the chair, just before it reached me.

Chris: *What was that all about? Why did she react that way?*

Me: Amy had read something on the internet about a rare insect that looks like an ordinary ladybird. It's beginning to be found in the UK and is, in fact, a deadly, poisonous creature, one bite from which would finish someone off within moments.

Apparently, that particular arrangement of spots gave this one away as the deadly mock-ladybird that needed to be treated with the respect we would give to a tarantula. Amy had identified it - but I had no idea. I'd never heard of such a thing.

As soon as she explained, Amy's reaction made total sense. Rather than being annoyed or puzzled, rather than protesting, I was eternally grateful for her intervention.

Chris: *And what happened to the deadly insect?*

Me: No need to worry. There wasn't one. It was all fiction. I don't know anyone called Amy. It was just to illustrate my point.

Chris: *Ok so what was the point?*

Me: Amy warned me of the danger. I ignored her so she got agitated, raised her voice and then got up and knocked my hand away. At first I was puzzled and then I was grateful.

Chris: *Her response escalated, like my fear of driving turning into a full panic attack?*

Me: Yes it's similar. So why did I change my reaction?

Chris: *You found out why she did it.*

Me: Yes that's right. That detail, that tiny piece of information made all the difference. Without it, it seemed like Amy was acting irrationally. Knowing that detail makes it all make sense.

And Amy could be right or wrong. She could have actually saved my life. Alternatively, she could have miscounted the spots on that tiny creature or she could have been misinformed. In one way, on one level, it doesn't actually matter whether she was right or not. What matters is that she was acting in my best interest. She was acting like my best friend.

Having my hand batted away from something that I had assumed was a cute and familiar black and red creature, by someone who is a life-long friend and ally, now has a logical explanation. Whether she was right or wrong, whether she was sure or just suspected that I was in danger, she still did the right thing based on the best information she had at the time.

If it later emerged that she had been wrong all along, that she had misunderstood what she'd been told, or maybe had relied on an expert who had not given her the full story, I'd still be grateful that she had acted like a true friend.

Chris: *So are you saying that my subconscious could be keeping me from driving to keep me safe? Could it believe I've got something that might make driving dangerous for me, like epilepsy or heart disease that could lead to me losing control of the car?*

Me: Possibly. But that's just one of several likely - and dozens of extremely unlikely but also possible explanations. And my job is to ask Amy and encourage her to lead me to the information that will resolve the puzzle.

Chris: *And what makes you think the subconscious mind is really like Amy? Is it really our best friend?*

Me: What controls us? What causes things to happen within us? Let's start with the physical side of us. What causes our heart to beat? What causes our digestive system to process what we've eaten? What causes us to blink or sneeze?

Chris: *Pat went through all that stuff with me. I know the answer. It's the subconscious mind.*

Me: That's right – and if something happens within us, then something must have caused it to happen. Something must be in the driving seat. Something must be orchestrating this remarkable self-adjusting, highly functional being to enable it to achieve all it does.

Scientists have worked for decades to create artificial limbs that work with some of the dexterity of the human hand. But they haven't added the beauty. They haven't captured the subtle sensitivity that allows the owner to feel the warmth and affection of the touch from a friend, a parent or a lover. They haven't managed to replicate the complexity and the soul that the concert pianist transmits through their hands and fingers, through their whole body, into the piano to create the music that can so move and transfix an audience with its emotion.

Chris: *No - I agree.*

Me: And the computer that controls that artificial limb does just that. If the heart or the kidney or the lungs also needed artificial aid, then a separate computer would be needed for each. And if those functions needed to be co-ordinated, then there would need to be even more power and complexity in the system.

Chris: *What do you mean?*

Me: When we drive a car with a manual gearbox, we need to press the clutch before we move the gear lever, and we need to control the clutch based partly on the tone of the engine noise as it reaches its biting point, and we need to be able to do that while watching the road and waiting for an opportunity to pull out into fast moving traffic.

Chris: *Ok I get it.*

Me: And while all that is going on, the kids in the back are starting to make a lot of noise. They could simply be being kids and displaying high spirits. Or it could be that one of them has just swallowed a peanut and is choking.

No worries, it was just high spirits.

Chris: *Phew – I was there!!!*

Me: So are you beginning to get the picture of just how powerful is that computer that is our life-support system, that enables all those physical parts of us to work, to co-ordinate with each other?

Chris: *Yes – it's pretty amazing.*

Me: And there's more. While all of that is going on, the digestive system has detected the chemical composition of the food that's been eaten, the food that is now in the stomach. It has analysed it and worked out the best kind of digestive juices for the most efficient and effective processing of that mix of food. It then causes the various organs to produce those juices and to deliver them to the stomach. Some foods are best digested with some kinds of juices, some with others. It may be better, as some nutritionists advise, to separate out the food we eat so that the proteins and carbohydrates are eaten at different times. That would make it so much easier for our computer.

Chris: *My Aunty Kitty has just gone on that diet and is feeling loads better now.*

Me: Yes, lots of people have, but most of us manage to eat a whole variety of different kinds of foods from all the different food groups, in the same meal, without indigestion, without any undue difficulty or discomfort. Our computer just gets on with it.

Chris: *Not another computer analogy...*

Me: No, it's ok, this time I feel an episode of a soap coming on.

Just a minute! An emergency! Sally is in the middle of a traffic jam and her son has gone into anaphylactic shock. She has a mobile phone and can ring for an ambulance, but A&E is just a few hundred yards away and her child's life is hanging by a thread. Her subconscious quickly assesses, with the help of some conscious thought and some decision-making, that the best chance of saving his life is to pick him up and carry him those few hundred yards.

That is far, far more than her body is normally asked to do on a daily basis – so she's going to need to call in the cavalry. All leave is cancelled. Everyone is on red-alert. That digestive process is one of the first to get moth-balled. It is simply switched off. All that blood and oxygen, all those nutrients that the digestive process would have used are now needed urgently. It's a matter of life and death.

The digestive system is switched off temporarily and all those resources, and any other resources that can be diverted, are poured into the muscles of the heart and lungs, the arms and legs, the brain, the hearing and sight. Everything is focussed as much as is possible while keeping Sally alive, on getting her son to A&E for that urgent life-saving treatment.

Only once the child is handed over and the medics have stabilised his condition will the parent's body begin to return from red-alert to slightly more normal functioning.

Chris: *What kind of computer could do all that?*

Me: I don't believe there is one outside of science-fiction that could come anywhere near that.

And it all just happens automatically. In such emergency situations, all the person is consciously aware of is the small number of choices that they need to make. Do they ring and wait for the ambulance? Do they get the child out and run the rest of the way? What would get them there the quickest?

In normal circumstances, a person of small stature that rarely takes part in physical activity of any kind of strenuous nature would not even consider that they had the strength and stamina to run such a distance carrying the weight of a young child. But that thought doesn't cross the parent's mind. The subconscious mind has taken over and made the impossible actually happen. In my estimation, it has worked a miracle.

Chris: *And that's all because I asked if the subconscious was like Amy.*

Me: So what do you think? Is it?

Chris: *Maybe it is, but maybe it's far, far more. What you've described, and I've heard stories of similar super-human feats of life-saving in real life – so maybe it's more like some cartoon super-hero.*

So if it's that clever, that resourceful, that powerful, how could it possibly ever go wrong?

Me: I feel a 'once upon a time' moment coming on.

Chris: *Oh for goodness sake....*

Big sister

Me: Let me introduce you to my big sister, Ellie. She is just a few years older than me, and is a very caring, nurturing person. When we were very young, she used to walk to school with me, made sure I wore my coat when it was cold and wet, helped me with my homework and fought my battles for me in the playground. The list was endless.

She recognised my small frame, my lack of experience, my sensitivity to conflict and frustration and used all her extra strengths in all those areas to smooth my passage through those early years in the big wide world.

She was doing everything with the best of intentions. She loved me – and still does. I'm her kid sister and she has known me since those very first hours and days of my life. She became my self-appointed guardian, happy to be able to help.

Chris: *She sounds great – I wish I'd had a sister like that.*

Me: Wait until you hear the whole story. What she didn't know then, what she hadn't yet had chance to learn, was that the more she cared for me in that way, the more she did things for me, the less I was able to grow and develop. She was actually causing me to be the weak and needy child that she mistakenly believed I already was.

Chris: *I'm not sure I understand.*

Me: I needed to fall and graze my knees to know that they heal. I needed to hear other kids call me names so I could see that no bones got broken that way and I could think of suitable replies of my own. I needed to get my homework wrong so I could learn from my mistakes, gain my own understanding, my own way of coping and living – just as she had done.

Chris: *Ok, I see it now.*

Me: The more she 'helped' me, the less I developed and the more I started to actually need her help. Then she felt justified in her assessment of my capabilities and doubled her efforts to transform all of life's tropical storms into the occasional mild shower.

But actually, other than being younger than her, I was the same size as she had been at my age. I was just as clever and capable as she had been at my age – but she couldn't remember that. She was still very young herself at that time.

And as she grew and matured, she became even cleverer and more resourceful and more devious in her methods so as to allow me some dignity in my neediness. She learnt how to discretely cut up my food or fasten my shoes for me when no one was looking. She found so many ways to hide her interventions by giving them some kind of validation that no-one would think to question.

Chris: *That doesn't sound good, but presumably it got resolved somehow. How did things get sorted out?*

Me: She couldn't resolve it all by herself. She needed a bit of help from outside. One day, Dad took her to one side and had a quiet word in her ear. He explained all that stuff that Ellie was too young to understand. It was hard for her to learn that she had been creating my handicaps, had been hindering me with her kindness. At first, she resisted, she denied, she put her fingers in her ears and sang la-la-la. She loved me so much. She couldn't bear to think that she might have actually been getting in my way with all that she had been doing.

But steadily, with gentle perseverance, Dad gradually helped her to understand and to learn how to step back in a way that would best help me to catch up all that missed learning. She slowly and gently withdrew, just a bit at a time, and watched to see how I got on. It was hard, at first, for her to watch me wobble, to take those first scary and wavering steps, but she saw me graze my knees, cry, clean and dress my wounds and get back out there – and she was so proud of me.

Chris: *So do you guys get on ok now? Did you both get over it?*

Me: If you re-wind a bit, you get to the bit where I mentioned a 'once upon a time' moment. She's not really my sister. I haven't actually got a sister.

Chris: *So remind me – what's this story about? Is she your subconscious mind as well?*

Me: Yes - she's my personal assistant, by best friend and my big sister all rolled into one – and the rest! She's that wonderful, endlessly watchful, caring and nurturing but also strict and fair, that fantastically powerful hidden part of my mind. She's that amazing part of the mind that each and every one of us has. Without her or him, we would be nothing like the wonderful creatures that we are and can grow into. When we really were so young and defenceless, she never did let us down. And she never knowingly or intentionally will.

Chris: *So why does she sometimes cause us problems?*

Me: Sometimes, in some ways, on some issues, she is capable of misjudging, maybe underestimating, our qualities, our potential, our spirit. She sometimes bases her judgement on assessments made before she was old enough to see us in a true perspective. And having made some of her judgements, she's too busy watching out for us day by day to go back and reassess. And just like when she adds up a column of figures and makes 9+7=15, when she gets to that same point again in her re-checking, she calls it 15 again.

Chris: Until Dad steps in.

   Me: Yes and Dad is really an LCH therapist. He can look at that column of figures with a fresh point of view. He can proof-read that huge subconscious-user-guide and find that typo or that inconsistency or ambiguity. He can check all the most important details for accuracy and easily replace that 15 with 16. Then he can help along and guide the process of reworking all those following calculations until every after-effect of that original error has been put right.

And from then on, our upgraded, fine-tuned, much wiser subconscious only helps us when we need it. She continues to take over the routine tasks so we can concentrate on the new and interesting challenges. She lets us learn all those essential lessons and only takes over once we've mastered those tasks.

She just needed someone to shine a torch on the path and point out the loose stone. She's so keen to have another look if she knows that all her best intentions are understood and recognised and appreciated. She's so quick to correct those tiny details that slipped under her radar when she was very young and also too busy being hyper-vigilant on our behalf.

Chris: The more I learn about my big sister, the more I like her.

   Me: Me too!

First aid

Chris: *I get it now – she got it wrong because she was just as young as we were at the time – but why didn't she correct it when she learnt more and became more experienced? If the subconscious mind has our best interests at heart, and is as powerful and clever as you believe, how can it be that it doesn't go back and sort out these errors? If it wants to do what's best for us and has so much processing power, so much multitasking capability, how could it possibly be that the subconscious mind could ever need the help of a therapist? Can you illustrate that one for me?*

Me: Picture the subconscious mind as an elderly relative. A young child, Susie, is being looked after by her very loving and capable aged greatgrandpa. No-one doubts for a moment that great grandpa's intentions are 100% for Susie's best interest. We also know that he has behind him the knowledge and experience from bringing up his own children and from helping bring up his children's children. He is fit and well and alert and competent - well-equipped in all ways for the job in hand.

9 7

Chris: *Is this another episode of that soap?*

Me: That's right. Susie suddenly has an accident while playing with a new toy. She has cut herself on a sharp piece of plastic that broke because she was trying to stand on it to reach up to the shelf for some chocolate biscuits. It's been a long time since great-grandpa had to call on his knowledge of first aid. The last time he did, the treatment for a burn was to put butter on it, and the routine treatment for a bleeding wound was a tourniquet, a grazed knee was cleaned with iodine.

Chris: *Ok I get that. Best practice in first aid keeps changing - we get better and better as we analyse what works and what doesn't. I'm a keen First Aider attached to a volunteer group and I'm regularly on duty at football matches and concerts – so I would expect to keep bang up to date with the latest advice. We expect the less experienced first aiders, the ones that do a refresher every few years, to pick things up as best they can and update whenever they hear of some new and safer procedure.*

Me: Great grandpa tried to put a tourniquet round Susie's arm to stop the bleeding from that cut on her hand, and tied it so tight that it did in fact stop the bleeding from the cut, but it did that by cutting off the blood supply to the whole of the lower arm and hand. Susie complained that it hurt and was told, "I know it hurts but we have to stop that bleeding. It's for your own good."

The great-grandpa is relieved now, the bleeding has stopped and all is under control and can wait until Susie's parents get home from work in a few hours if only Susie will stop complaining that her arm is hurting even more.

Chris: *I'm ahead of you – this is scary!*

Me: That loving aged relative has no idea that his well-meaning and well thought out intervention could end in permanent damage to Susie's hand and arm. And far, far worse than that - once that tourniquet has been in place for more than about 15 minutes, she will be in the same potentially fatal situation as the victim of a crush injury. If the aged relative or the returning parents then remove that tourniquet - without medical treatment Susie could be poisoned by the toxins that have built up behind that circulation-stopping bandage.

Chris: *And all while great grandpa was doing what he believed was best for Susie!*

But what point are you making here?

Me: Well you're the first aid expert here, so what was the cause of this dangerous development from a simple minor cut from an accident?

Chris: *Great grandpa was acting on some information that many people believed was good first aid practice many years ago. He hadn't heard that that advice had been updated, hadn't learnt how dangerous such treatment could be. He probably hadn't been in a situation where he needed to use that kind of first-aid, probably hadn't had any reason to ask, to question what he'd learnt decades previously, and hadn't heard about any harm that technique had caused.*

Me: And the remedy?

Chris: *He just needed a bit of information, needed to have it explained to him that what he was aiming to achieve, to stop the loss of blood, would be better done using a different technique. Once he had that update, Susie would be in much safer hands.*

But again, what's that got to do with the subconscious mind and LCH?

Me: It's the answer to how something as powerful and as well-meaning as the subconscious mind could get things so totally wrong. We don't tend to revisit old information unless we get a clue or a lesson that tells us it might be worth checking a bit more thoroughly.

Chris: *Ok, I get it. The subconscious probably does the same as the great grandpa did, and relies on old information – doesn't even question it for a moment, just assumes it's correct – but it might be out of date. Is that it?*

Me: Yes, that's what I believe and what seems to be confirmed by the treatments I've given, the information I've received and the outcomes that patients have described.

Chris: *My friend has a severe allergy and has to be really careful around peanuts as taking in even the tiniest quantity could send her into anaphylactic shock. If the subconscious mind works as you believe it does, could you explain what's going on there? How is it that the body works so hard at keeping us healthy and comfortable, keeping us warm by shivering when the temperature drops, keeping us cool by sweating when it rises, developing antibodies to infections and viruses and bacteria so they can't make us so ill a second time – and yet goes into a tail-spin which can be fatal without rapid and targeted medication, as a result of a single peanut or a bee sting?*

Me: I don't think anyone knows anything for certain – and I certainly don't – but I'll describe what I believe could be happening. Imagine if, for some reason, in some circumstance, some combination of a whole heap of rare occurrences, the body's life-support system suddenly decided that the correction for a high body temperature was to shiver. It would respond to a very slight increase by starting the shivering response. That shivering response would, in fact, cause the temperature to rise even higher. The response would then be even more shivering – and so on.... What would be the result of that?

Chris: *It wouldn't be long before the person would be in extreme danger of major organ failure and eventually, if it wasn't corrected, they would die. But how could that happen?*

Me: Think of a fairly complex computer program that deals with numerous different circumstances, providing the appropriate response to each situation. It has been thoroughly tested from every angle that the developer and tester could devise. But there is no way of knowing if all eventualities have been covered by that testing. A particular set of circumstances that, individually, were never expected to happen, all happened at once, and that program goes off into a part of the processing that hasn't been tested – and it contains an error!

Chris: *Yes that's possible. But what's that got to do with the subconscious.*

Me: The subconscious mind is trying to help, but isn't aware that some information it has, and is relying on, is totally unquestioning of, may actually be out-of-date, no longer relevant, or never was relevant but was accepted at the time without question.

That's why most people who develop symptoms, conditions and issues requiring some kind of treatment had the best, most nurturing, most well-intended family circumstances. If Dad is always shouting, Mum is always drunk, then we learn pretty quickly that what they say and do is likely to have nothing to do with any kind of sense or reason. If Mum always looks after us, takes care of us, helps us in every kind of way, then we are likely to believe, until we learn otherwise, at a much older age, that everything she says and does is right, correct, the truth. And we may later end up relying on that

information to take us off along some cliff-edge
path that isn't safe, is full of potholes, is likely
to fall into the sea at any moment.

In my practice, most of the information that
turns out to be less than accurate tends to have
been gained within the first 10 or 15 years of
life. At that kind of age, we behave like sponges,
soaking up all we experience and trusting that
all we see and hear, especially from adults, from
well-meaning, caring, parents and friends of the
family, is 100% reliable. As we grow older, we
start learning to think and analyze before we
store any new information, and given the
appropriate reminder, we might just go back
and sanity-check some pre-analysis 'facts'. But
if we don't have the right experiences, the odd
stray and invalid line of code can easily lie
dormant and waiting to jump up and bite us if
we wander into some unfamiliar territory.

I only learnt that thunder wasn't caused by
clouds banging together and lightening wasn't
the resulting spark from that dramatic collision
in the sky when, at the tender age of 7, I
explained it back to one smirking brother while
the other, who had fed me the line in the first
place was happily sniggering in the corner.

I was 15 before I learnt that cider was alcoholic.
It was on the table in my pre-teen years with the
Tizer and the Irn-Bru at Sunday dinner, to go
with the roast beef and Yorkshire puddings, and
my parents had trusted that I wouldn't like the

taste so they wouldn't need to tell me not to drink it. I learnt at 15 because you were allowed to go in pubs at that age as long as you stuck to soft drinks. My school friends were quite sophisticated and were debating over whether they'd get away with it. I thought I'd play safe with some of that apple pop.

Chris: *Doh... I was almost thinking about asking you for treatment – but now I think I'll look elsewhere.*

Me: Hmmmm... maybe I should have kept quiet about that stuff. But seriously, it's all the experiences that I've had, all the misunderstandings that I've corrected for myself that have helped me to see how the subconscious mind could interpret something - and then rely on its interpretation – and then experience something that shows up some error – and then correct it. I believe that studying those kinds of situations helps me do my job better. It helps me understand more about the subconscious mind so I can work with it more effectively.

Chris: *It's ok – I've been talking to a few people recently who've had successful treatment from you, so you must be doing something right.*

Me: Thanks!

Reference library

Chris: *Ok so my fear of driving, then. There could be some information, some error that my subconscious mind has, that is causing it to give me that fear and make me want to avoid driving. So how do you get that information?*

Me: Have you ever done a crossword or a quiz, or tried to think who sang that song or which team won that sporting event - and just knew that you knew the answer, but however hard you tried, the answer just wouldn't come?

Chris: *Yes – often.*

Me: And you eventually learnt that as long as you kept on wracking your brains, demanding to know, there's no way that that information ever emerged.

Chris: *That's right. It's only when I finally give up and get on with other things that the answer ever arrives. So I learned to give up trying and say, 'it'll come to me' – and it usually does.*

Me: Yes, maybe it's minutes or hours later, maybe it's days, weeks or even months later, but sure enough, at some time after we give up trying to think of it, the answer pops into our mind, as if from nowhere.

If I asked you about something that happened to you earlier on today, even if it was quite a small detail like what time you had breakfast or what you ate for lunch, I'm guessing you'd be able to tell me.

Chris: *Probably.*

Me: And if I asked you about something that happened many years ago, but was a fairly big factor in a fairly memorable occasion, I'm guessing you'd probably be able to think and retrieve that information from your memory banks.

Chris: *Yes, again probably.*

Me: But what if I asked you what the weather was like on 30th May when you were 3 years old, then unless that particular date had some major significance for you and the weather was part of that significance, and as I've known you for at least 10 years, so, young as you look, you must be at least 15 by now, I'm pretty confident that you wont actually be able to remember - however hard you try.

Chris: *I agree - so how do you find it? How do you get that information? I feel another of your illustrations coming on...*

Me: Imagine a reference library with 2 types of department. The first is the one where you can wander in, use the index, find a book, take it off the shelf and read it to find the information you're after. Any information that is quite easy to get at by simply thinking, mentally looking for it, you could imagine as being the information stored in all of those books in that open reference library. Sometimes you have to give it a bit of time, work your way towards it. For example, what year did so-and-so win such-and-such a competition? Well you can't actually remember but you know you were doing that summer job at the bakery at the time, and that was just before you went to the 6th Form College, so it must have been 1983, right?

Chris: *Yes I'd do something like that if I could. It often helps.*

Me: You can follow clues, use the various indexes, by title, by author, by genre – and if enough of the right kinds of indexes exist, enough big landmark events were around at the time to help you get your bearings, you'll eventually find the information.

And if the information that would unlock the mystery of that unwanted symptom or condition or issue were to be found by that route, then you would find it and put it right for yourself. You wouldn't need any help. If you have any kind of problem, anything unpleasant, uncomfortable or worrying, then I'm sure you've gone through everything you can think of yourself, tried anything that sounded promising, and only given up and gone for help when you'd tried all avenues that you could find.

Chris: *Yes I've remembered the bus skidding but I can't seem to get over it. And I can't remember anything else that might be relevant.*

Me: Now imagine the kind of reference library where they won't let you in. Maybe the books are too rare and valuable or too fragile to let members of the public handle them. Or maybe there are just so many of them that even if they would let you in, that even if you searched for several lifetimes, you'd have very little chance of finding what you're after. You'd need to be a specialist in that field to have a reasonable chance of locating the fact you're looking for within any kind of reasonable time frame.

So they won't let you in, but instead they have provided some expert librarians to attend to your queries. All you need to do is go up to the desk and ask your question, and you might be told to take a seat, go and get a coffee, come back after lunch or go home and they will ring or email when they've got the response.

So going back to that crossword, that quiz, the elusive singer of that song. Imagine going to that desk, asking your question, watching the librarian set off into the depths of the archives and then, before they've even arrived at the index, you call them back saying, 'have you found it yet?', 'what's the answer?', 'I know it's there, have you looked under A,B or C?' You keep doing that and they're never going to get chance to search in their own way, use their own specialist skills, their own professional indexing system. You'll be getting in their way, slowing them down – trying to be helpful but actually making matters worse.

Chris: *So that's why trying to remember never works, then?*

Me: Yes – you would be getting in the way of the expert who knows how to search and how to know when they've found the answer.

Chris: *And how does that relate to your patients?*

Me: In treatment, we're looking for a tiny snapshot, a snippet of information from any time in the patient's life. So it's more likely to be in that reference library that needs the expert to search in. Before the patient came to us for treatment, they would have gone through everything they could think of, and might have found lots of relevant information, might even have seen it differently, got it back into perspective, but still the problem or symptom persists. So the patient has already fully and thoroughly searched that department where you can wander around and take books off the shelves. So there's no point in looking in that room any more. If it had been there, they would have found it, they would have fixed the dilemma, they would have got rid of the symptom.

So the information must be in the department with the librarian at the desk, waiting to do the searching for you. And to get that information, we need the patient to do the mental equivalent of going for a coffee or coming back after lunch so that we can get on with the job we've been trained to do in the quickest and most efficient manner.

So part of what is involved in treatment is taking the patient step-by-step to the point where they automatically drop off their request at the desk and then wait for that email to drop into their inbox.

Can you cope with a computer analogy?

Chris: *Go on – as long as it's not too complicated.*

Me: Your computer is broken and someone is trying to fix it for you. I guess you're not very technically minded so you need to rely on an expert.

Chris: *Right!*

Me: The person who has their hands on or even inside your computer is trying to fix it using some expert help from the manufacturer's telephone help-line. But the phone is too far away from the computer and it isn't a cordless one. Go on, let your imagination take you back to such days if you're way past all that now.

So your friendly local PC expert needs to ask the manufacturer's trouble-shooting expert a question. They ask you. You pass it on. The help-desk reply comes back to you. You pass it back to your local guy. If you do any kind of paraphrasing, any amendment, any rewording of any of those technical messages in either direction, what chance have you got of actually getting your PC fixed?

Chris: *None at all. I'd be bound to get it wrong.*

Me: You've certainly got the best chance if you disengage brain and simply act as a mechanical voicemail machine, passing on, word for word, matching the emphasis, keeping the whole of that information as true to what you received as is humanly possible.

Chris: *I get the point, but you've done all the training and it sounds like your patients need special skills too.*

Me: You might guess that we have a way of making that incredibly easy for the patient to do.

Chris: *Well I hope so, because I'm considering having treatment.*

Me: There's no need to wonder whether you'll be able to pass on the messages accurately – we take you through it step by step and we have tried and tested methods that have worked for so many people.

Chris: *But what if it doesn't work for me?*

Me: That's quite a common worry. People come for treatment for all sorts of symptoms and conditions and wrapped up in all of that is often a feeling that they'll be the one it doesn't work for, or the one that won't be able to do what's required.

Chris: *Yes, that's me on both counts.*

Me: If we ever find someone it doesn't work for, and that's pretty rare these days, we deal with it. LCH therapists are investigative therapists. We do this kind of work because we like thinking. We are problem-solvers, like puzzle-addicts, so if you present us with a new challenge, we'll be up for it and if necessary, put our collective powerful heads/brains/minds together to come up with a way that works for you.

Chris: *Pat's considering training. Will Pat be able to do all that stuff?*

Me: Yes – there's a full and varied training program that helps people to learn in their own way. All will be revealed in a step-by-step process that, as long as the student likes thinking, using logic, working things out, they'll learn and develop until they are part of that ever-growing band of Columbo-style hypnotherapists who will continue asking about 'just one more thing' until all pieces of the jigsaw are in place and that rogue piece of information is uncovered and put right.

Chris: *Are dirty raincoats and cigars compulsory?*

Me: Doh!

Symptom problem

Chris had had enough by then, and gone off to catch the bus, but was already wondering how to get the car back from the teenage son who was 'looking after it'.

Pat had got some information from the training school and came back with some more questions. I like questions....

Pat: *What would it take to get the subconscious mind to give you that information? Do you need to persuade it that that would be a good idea?*

Me: Remember that it's there to look after us, and it was saying, "I know it hurts but it's for your own good."

Pat: *So how do you encourage the subconscious mind to work with you? Do you have to work at it?*

Me: The patient arrives and tells me what they want treatment for. They want to get rid of something. They want something to change in some way. Whatever it is, it's causing them a problem. They wouldn't be spending their time and money otherwise.

And the person doing the speaking is being driven at that point by the conscious mind.

Pat: *Yes - we normally think before we speak. That's what we're taught from a very early age.*

Me: But in order to resolve the issue, to have any chance of helping the patient get rid of what their conscious mind sees as a problem, we need the help of that other part of their mind – the subconscious mind - the part that created what their conscious mind sees as a problem.

But the subconscious mind is designed to keep us well and safe and happy. It's not in the business of creating problems. Its job is to create solutions.

So what the conscious mind sees as a problem, the subconscious mind sees as a solution. And if we refer the conscious mind to the Solution of their fear of spiders, they're not likely to come back for session 2. They're going to seriously doubt our ability to help them if we imply that we see a fear of spiders as a Solution.

Equally, if we refer the subconscious mind to the Problem of their fear of spiders, the subconscious mind may develop a few colds or stomach upsets to cancel the booked appointments and not be too quick at providing reminders to re-book after that. Either that, or the patient will turn up but the answers may not be very forthcoming.

The subconscious mind can weigh up all our subconscious reassurance against that 'Problem' word and decide that it's not convinced that the therapist has any idea what the subconscious is designed for. It may decide that it's not in safe hands.

As the subconscious is listening all the time, not just during hypnosis, it's worth finding a few generic words for whatever is the specific 'thing to be treated'. Maybe Symptom, Condition, Issue or something a bit more focussed if appropriate, like Habit or Tendency or...... a thesaurus would come in handy here. We're looking for something both parts of the mind can see as a fact or a description without any implied value judgement.

And we need to also beware of expressions like 'over-weight', 'excess weight'. It's not excessive to the subconscious. It's exactly the right weight according to the subconscious. It's the weight that the subconscious chose and caused to be maintained. So maybe 'more weight than you consciously wish for', or something a bit more factual, 'more than x% body fat'...

Pat: *It's getting complicated – example please.*

Me: Fred has a problem. He hates smelly cheese and he lives with someone, Charlie, who can't live without it – who is only happy when the fridge, the kitchen, the whole house reeks of the stuff.

Fred asks Charlie to give it up - he gets on at Charlie, nags, begs and yells at Charlie, but Charlie won't budge. So Fred drags him along to an LCH therapist and all 3 are very happy because the plan is to look at why Charlie is so keen on smelly cheese so that this disagreement can be resolved.

Charlie is particularly happy because the therapist keeps stressing that treatment isn't about making

Charlie give up his smelly cheese – just find out why he needs it so much – and if it emerges that he does really need it, then nothing will change. Fred will then understand and accept that Charlie needs it and stop nagging him. If it emerges that he doesn't need it any more, though, then he'll be able to easily give it up for himself – but no-one's going to take it away from him!

And then treatment starts with "so this Problem that you have with smelly cheese". Fred is happy, someone understands him - smelly cheese is a Problem.

But Charlie loves his smelly cheese and just wants to be left alone to enjoy it in peace. When he hears it referred to as a 'Problem', he feels misunderstood. He decides that he's been tricked by Fred and the therapist - and there's no way he's joining in with treatment.

Whenever he hears that word 'Problem', whenever it's said to Fred and he overhears, and when it's said directly to him when Fred is out of earshot, all that reassurance that the therapist gave him turns into empty promises. Problems are things to be got rid of. No-one wants a Problem.

The therapist sees the way Charlie winces each time he says that 'P' word and begins to look at the 'P' word from Charlie's point of view and sees why. So he looks for a way of removing That Word from his treatment. He starts referring to the smelly cheese dilemma in a way he hopes that both Fred and Charlie will understand and be comfortable with.

Fred drags Charlie along for another session with the therapist. Charlie braces himself for the 'P' word but it never comes. The therapist says things like, 'these cravings for smelly cheese', 'this habit of choosing the smellier cheeses', and even, 'the cheeses that Charlie prefers but Fred dislikes'.

Fred and Charlie both feel understood and valued for their different wants and needs. They continue with treatment and all finally gets resolved. Fred mysteriously develops a taste for slightly more adventurous morsels from the deli.

Pat: *Very amusing, but I could do with a more realistic example if you can manage it please.*

Symptom friend

Me: We can assume that our symptom or condition or issue is a problem. In fact, we're unlikely to look at it in any other way. It's unwanted, unhealthy, uncomfortable or painful or agonising, it's worrying, inconvenient, embarrassing – so calling it a problem is putting it mildly. But there are a few examples that can illustrate to us that symptoms can be there to help us.

For example, if we didn't get toothache when there was decay in a tooth, then we wouldn't have any reason to go to the dentist. If we didn't go to the dentist, then the decay could spread until the whole tooth broke up and fell out. The decay could spread to other teeth and even the jaw. We could end up unable to eat and speak properly.

Leprosy is a classic example of a disease that shows just how important are the messages we get that tell us before we do any damage to ourselves. The sufferers don't know that what they are doing is damaging skin and bone. They feel no sensations, they get no feedback to help them stay safe and healthy.

High blood pressure is known as the silent killer because the person affected rarely feels any helpful warning signs such as pain or discomfort or fatigue. The first sign of the condition could be the fatal or debilitating heart-attack or stroke. The damage is happening in the background, without making its presence felt, without giving us a chance to take remedial action. That could be one of the reasons that doctors take almost every opportunity to test it for us.

Angina is also helpful in that it warns the sufferer and insists they rest. The pain of a heart attack is different. That is the pain of damage already done, whereas angina forces us to stop and rest so that damage is less likely to occur.

The pain of a broken arm is very specific. It causes us to support the arm and keep it still and hold it at right-angles against the body. The pain is at its mildest if we comply. Any deviation from that is rewarded by a sharp and attention-grabbing stabbing sensation. The pain is helping us to minimise the risk of further damage and to promote the most rapid and effective healing.

Pat: *Ok I get that the symptom can be useful – it has a purpose.*

Me: And there are various other phenomena that seem to hint that this is more the rule than the exception. Have you ever had toothache, reluctantly made that dentist appointment and then happily found that the pain went away?

Pat: *Yes. It was bizarre. I cancelled the appointment on the assumption that whatever it was that caused the pain must have gone away, but then the pain came back.*

Me: It's a fairly well known pattern. And it reminds me of the way the average caring Mum would behave.

"Have you made that appointment yet?" "I forgot. I'll do it tomorrow"

"No you won't – you'll do it now!" "Aw but Mum..."

"None of your Aw but's – DO IT NOW!" "Ok"

"Have you done it?" "Yes"

Silence for a week....

"Have you been to the dentist?" "No, I cancelled it because I had a football match."

"Ok that's it – I'm making that appointment for you and I'm going to take you there myself!"

So it seems to make sense now. The subconscious tells us when we need to do something, to take care of something, to get some help. It makes the message fit the urgency of the need. If we have a grumbling minor ache, we can make an appointment for sometime next week when we're not so busy. If the ache becomes more constant and more severe, we'll book in at the first opportunity and cancel other arrangements. If we try to ignore it, it stops us in our tracks and forces us to be dependent on others to take us to A&E.

There are many examples of people successfully using self-hypnosis to silence the pain of a dental or surgical procedure. If someone cuts our skin, that's normally something that we should be trying to prevent. Self-hypnosis can work by the individual explaining to their subconscious mind that this is a medical intervention designed to improve their health and well-being, so the pain is not necessary.

Pat: *So are you saying that pain isn't actually a physical or biological consequence of the messages received by the nerve endings? You seem to be inferring that it's the subconscious mind that translates those messages into pain if it believes that that pain is needed to prompt us to take defensive action.*

Me: It makes sense to me to look at it that way.

Pat: *So could it actually be that all symptoms, conditions and issues are there to help us? Would it be a good idea to treat them all like that smoke alarm and take appropriate action, check what set it off, leave the building, or whatever was the safest response before thinking about silencing it?*

Me: On the whole, yes, I think so. But then, I would say that, wouldn't I?

Pat: *Yes and all those examples are of symptoms that we can recognise. If we have a pain following an illness or injury, then we know why there's a pain. We want the pain to go away and we may take pain-killers, but we know the pain won't fully go until the damage or disease has fully healed.*

But what about when there's no obvious cause? We don't know why it hurts - there's no sign of a physical cause, so we simply want the pain to go away.

Me: And yet we'd make sure the cause is treated if it was a fracture or a sprain or measles or chicken-pox.

Pat: *Of course. But there are loads of medical tests, many different signs and symptoms that our medical experts can use to determine the cause. When they all prove negative, when nothing physical can be detected, no blood chemical, no hormone level, not even a gene to explain it, why can't you just take the pain away?*

Me: I don't believe anything just happens for no reason. I just think we haven't developed all the necessary tests yet.

Pat: *I'd really like to have some more real-life examples*

Me: I can't give any real details about any genuine cases as that would break my patients' confidentiality, so instead I'll give you some works of fiction. They're based on the theory behind LCH and some details from various treatments I've given and received and otherwise learnt of – all mixed up.

Pat: *Ok. That will have to do. It's better than nothing.*

Symptom – excess weight and can't lose it

Me: And following the theme of, "if the subconscious were a person, what kind of person would it be?", she's female in this example because she's a mum. She's a nurturing, caring parent who often finds herself saying, "I know you don't want this medicine but it's for your own good". She also looks after quite young children who wouldn't understand that concept and so just does it anyway, without any explanation. She hides the bitterness of a vital medicine behind the welcome taste of something sweet. She distracts and otherwise amuses her young offspring just enough to allow all those vital tasks to be completed, to keep them safe, well fed, clean and happy.

My Mum is causing me to be overweight. I don't want to be thin, slim and elegant, size 0 like the imaginary air-brushed models on my magazine cover. I just want to be fairly average in size and shape so that I feel healthy and can buy clothes in the mainstream high-street outlets. But Mum knows best.

According to the medical weight charts, I'm definitely overweight and steadily creeping into the obese column. I try to eat healthily but when I do, mum turns down the thermostat so that the food I eat gets processed at an extremely low rate. This has 2 effects. One is that even if I never consume more than 1000 calories a day, my weight still increases. The other effect is that, as the food I'm eating isn't getting burned up at an average pace, I don't have enough fuel to be averagely active. I try to live my normal life but feel too tired to do more than the basic survival tasks.

Also, she distracts me when I'm in the supermarket so that I don't notice how many bars of chocolate, tubs of ice-cream and packets of biscuits she's put into my trolley. She hides them under the broccoli and the spinach. She specifically chooses the ones quite near their sell-by date. Then, when I get home, she points them out to me and tells me that I mustn't waste them. They need eating up before they go off and I can go on my diet after that.

And she talks to me, gets me engrossed in some interesting conversation, just as I go to the fridge for my salad and fish, and puts the ice-cream in my hand instead. And she continues to talk to me, ask me questions, gets me really engrossed in some debate while she puts a few extra spoonfuls of ice-cream on my dish. And this distraction continues until I've eaten a whole load, washed the dish and put it away. And she keeps up the banter until I've completely forgotten my loaded starter and set off, with a sense of purpose, to cook my healthy fish and prepare that salad which I can then eat and remember with a wonderful sense of pride and a feeling of accomplishment.

She then stands next to me in the morning and confirms that either the scales must be inaccurate or that I have the 'fat gene' - and it's so unfair!

Pat: *So why would your Mum, who loves you dearly, has been with you all your life, who wants only the best for you and would do anything to make you happy, why is she sabotaging your attempts to reduce from clinically obese to healthily average?*

Me: One of the effects of my obesity is that I can't find myself a partner. No-one wants to go out with me. It's pretty grim, but I console myself with the promise that this latest diet will work and then I'll be slim and attractive and that guy at the office will ask me out.

But Mum knows different. She knows that I'm kidding myself. She knows that because she created that idea, a little white lie, in the first place, and she did it to keep me happy.

Pat: *Keeping you happy... now this sounds a bit more like your Mum.*

Me: She knows that I'm ugly and will never find a partner, knows that no-one will ever want me, and she knows that I must never learn that painful truth – I would be devastated if I did. I would know that it was all about me, that no-one would ever want me, however slim I was, and I would have no hope of ever being happy.

While I believe that all will be ok as soon as I lose that extra couple of stone, I retain that hope and expectation of a happy and fulfilled life. I just have to find a diet that works!

And to keep me from learning that damning truth, Mum has to get in the way every time, so that I never have more that a week or two as a slim person before it all comes piling back on again. I can enjoy feeling good about myself for a couple of weeks. She wants me to be happy and optimistic and prepared to keep trying, but she won't let me stay slim long enough for me to expect and hope to meet someone and start a relationship.

So it's beginning to make some kind of warped sense. If I really am so ugly that no-one will want to look at me, then by making me fat and keeping me that way most of the time, Mum is actually making me happier than I would be if I ever learnt the whole truth. I'm unhappy as a fat person, but boy would I feel so much worse if I knew what Mum knew. I could hit the depths of despair and want to end my life-long prison sentence. I might even choose suicide as the better option, the lesser evil.

Pat: *No Mum would let that happen. So what could be going on with your Mum?*

Me: Just like the aged relative with the tourniquet, Mum could have got her wires crossed. She might actually be mistaken about my appearance, about what she sees as my false, mistaken expectations that one day I would be loved and be happy. She could be wrong about my fate of never getting the chance to enjoy life.

Pat: *Yes I agree she could easily be wrong – but how could she get that wrong idea in the first place?*

Me: Mum remembers loads of things that I've forgotten, and she can recall a day, many years ago, when I was just a toddler. She was always proud of me, always showing me off to friends and relatives, and was particularly keen that great-uncle Albert would agree that his great-niece was the best in every possible way. On that day, all those years ago, she was shocked to hear Albert proclaim to all and sundry that I looked "terrible". Albert had been away for many years and this was the first time he'd seen me. Mum was hanging on his every word and knew he was wise and well-travelled and had been around the most beautiful and charming women in the world, so Mum was expecting confirmation that I was up there with the best.

But Mum had forgotten that I was still suffering the after-effects of that allergic reaction to those antibiotics that had caused my face to swell up. It still hadn't settled back to normal but she'd just got used to seeing me that way. Albert wasn't saying I was ugly, he was commenting on how badly that illness had affected my looks. But Mum had misunderstood – and she was devastated.

From then on, she listened carefully to everything that everyone said about me, she watched everyone's reactions when they met me, and found a morsel to worry about on every occasion. She found a way to interpret every look, every word, every intonation, every bit of emphasis as confirming what Albert had said. After all, Albert was so wise, so kind, so clever that he must be right and something Aunty Edie said about my complexion could have been a criticism. And I didn't get to sit on the front row for the school photo, and I didn't get called up onto the stage at the panto last year...

And eventually, Mum stopped watching so carefully, stopped analysing every scrap of information, stopped collecting clues. She had enough. I was ugly! And she had to protect me from ever learning the truth.

And now, here come the cavalry to sort it all out...

With the benefit of LCH, Mum put a few extra facts together with those damning words and saw them for what they really were. She saw the whole thing in context, put it into perspective. Her precious daughter wasn't ugly after all, she had just been ill at the time and her appearance had shocked Albert into making that understandable, but unfortunately ambiguous remark. Once the more likely meaning, knowing Albert's kind personality and loving nature, had been offered to Mum, she was happy to throw out the old meaning.

She then had a look at some of those other bits of information. I wasn't on the front row of the school photo because I was quite tall for my age. And when Aunty Edie mentioned my complexion, I was a typical spotty teenager at the time. And at that panto, I was one of hundreds of children that also hadn't been called up onto the stage. One by one, they all got filed under 'more evidence that my daughter was just a typical kid at that age'.

So now Mum knows that I'm not ugly and so she can let me lose that weight without risking me looking in the mirror and then topping myself. She can let me eat when I'm hungry, stop when my stomach is full enough, eat a fairly balanced, healthy, nutritious diet and she has put the thermostat back up on the boiler so I can process the food, get back to the kind of life I always wanted, a fair week's work followed by a Friday night on the dance floor, Saturday round the town buying some new fashionable clothes and a Sunday walk with my new boyfriend and his rambling mates.

That's pretty much 'happy ever after'

And it is imaginary - but why not?

Pat: *Ok, but it's just one story. I need more than that but I have to go now. Chris will be here soon and we can swap stories next time we meet up.*

Symptom – poor response to kidney transplant

Chris: *Pat was in a rush so I guess you got carried away with your stories again. Go on, I'm sitting comfortably.*

Me: Sophie had been feeling ill for months, under the weather and steadily getting worse. Fatigue, lack of appetite, she felt terrible and couldn't do anything, so she went to the doctor who took a history, did some tests and referred her to a specialist as she suspected kidney failure. This suspicion was confirmed. Sophie had all the recommended treatment and her condition stabilised. She didn't feel quite how she used to, but it wasn't getting any worse and she could just about cope as long as she had her regular dialysis. Her husband and family needed to adjust to her suddenly increased dependence.

They put her on the kidney transplant waiting list, but weren't optimistic that there would be a cadaver donor within the next year or two. She knew that a successful transplant could give her back her pre-failure quality of life.

All her friends and relatives wanted to help, and all her blood relatives who were well enough to be considered were tested for compatibility with a view to a transplant from a live donor. No-one was a good enough match.

Her husband then offered to be a live donor. They had been married for 32 years and had a close and loving relationship, but he was only 53, and he would be taking various risks for the procedure itself and also then be relying on the remaining kidney to stay healthy and effective for the rest of his life. And even the best of marriages can fail, especially when there is some extra pressure on them, and this is one huge extra pressure.

They eventually agreed to go ahead. Her husband, the medical team and Sophie herself all decided that it was the best option. Her husband wanted his happy, healthy wife back and knew his love for her was strong enough. Sophie found herself accepting – feeling strangely puzzled by the whole affair, but giving her consent nevertheless.

The transplant went ahead and all went well with the procedure. Her husband recovered very quickly and so did Sophie. But then they found a problem. Her body began to reject his kidney in spite of the medication designed to suppress that rejection response, medication that normally works extremely well.

She was still alive but not much healthier than before the transplant.

She had a friend who studied LCH and had followed the course of her illness with intense interest and concern. He suggested Sophie investigate this therapy and she feared for his sanity. She couldn't imagine how hypnotherapy could stop her body from rejecting her husband's well-matched kidney. But she couldn't think of anything else and the medical team had no other suggestions up to then.

LCH is complementary, not alternative, so she didn't need to choose between the two types of treatment. The NHS was paying for her ongoing medical care and she could afford to have a weekly session, so she made an appointment and went along, feeling totally bemused - but her friend seems confident that this COULD help her. She had very little to lose and loads to gain. Not a difficult choice.

Her therapist took a full history, asking her all sorts of questions that didn't seem even vaguely relevant to her, and then reminded her that there was no external cause of her original kidney failure that anyone had been able to determine. For some reason, it had just failed. Then, she'd had a fairly poor response to the dialysis. Some people feel quite a bit better on that treatment than Sophie had. Then, although the operation had gone well and the kidney had been an extremely close match, and the anti-rejection drugs are normally powerful enough to allow a full and healthy post-transplant existence, she had still found herself feeling very poorly.

He suggested that there might be a pattern there, that she seemed to have become ill without there being any trauma or virus, bacteria or other externally originated cause – and that her response to each type of treatment has been at the poor end of the scale. This led to her remembering various other illnesses that she'd had in the past, and that pattern was always there – she was always slow to recover, needed the strongest treatment, needed the longest period of recuperation.

Chris: *So why was that?*

Me: He described all her medical treatment as being the essential bailing out to prevent her boat from sinking, and LCH as being an equally vital process of finding and fixing that hole so the water wouldn't keep on pouring in. That made sense to her and it meant that both could happen side by side. She wouldn't need to choose between them.

She had a number of sessions and was so tired and weary that she took him at his word and put her feet up, let herself get nicely relaxed and let him get on with his job. She didn't want him to explain it all to her, just tell her what he wanted her to do and she would trust him. Some people want to know all the details, she was no different normally, but at that point, she had no energy to spare for that. He was recommended by her friend, the first session had made her feel reassured and that feeling, although she couldn't have put her finger on why that was happening, that feeling of reassurance grew and grew.

After a few weekly sessions, she started to feel a little bit different – not much, just a bit more energy, a bit more motivation. A few more weekly sessions went by and then the therapist told her that he would see her again in a month's time because some progress had been made and it needed a little time to work through. She was to come back then to see how things were developing.

By the time she came back, the improvement had been so steady and consistent that she was feeling as well as the transplant team had originally predicted. The anti-rejection medication was doing its job and her energy level was getting closer and closer to her pre-failure level. She put her feet up and relaxed and let him get on with his work again, and at the end of the session, he was able to tell her that all his tests had had the desired outcome, that all traces of that hole in her boat had been well and truly sealed up. He wasn't expecting her to have any further problems and didn't need to arrange any more sessions, but if she had any concern in the future, then she could get in touch and he would be able to quickly and easily fix any tiny leaks that had been hidden by the main one.

It didn't make any sense to her, but she wasn't bothered. She felt so much better and wasn't going to waste any of her precious new energy on analysing it. She wanted to go on that holiday that she and her husband had been promising themselves for when she felt well enough to enjoy it.

Chris: *She might not want to know, but I do! Why was it causing her to be so ill, and why did it suddenly start letting her recover?*

Me: Sophie's subconscious mind had been looking after her in a strange and puzzling way, until you know the full story. When she was 5 years old, her mum had been carrying her, and her dad had been carrying her younger sister, then aged 3. They were wandering around the town, looking at the shops. It was December and they were choosing Christmas presents to put on their list for Santa. Being a typical December, it was very cold and she was enjoying the warmth from being carried by mum and it was quite a long shopping trip so she was happy not to have to walk.

Then her mum said, "You'll have to walk now, you're too heavy". Sophie found herself cold and unhappy as mum put her down to walk. She didn't believe she was too heavy because her mum and her dad were always trying to get her to eat all her dinner, and they wouldn't be doing that if she had been too heavy. Mum must have been lying. She had put her down for some other reason.

Then, when she went to school, she found herself getting left out of some of the games and didn't know why, but recognised the feeling as being similar to how she had felt when Mum had made her walk that day in town.

A couple of years later, her younger sister Beth got measles and everyone was looking after her, and forgetting about Sophie. And that familiar feeling returned. She found herself watching out for it, expecting it, seeing it coming and feeling that way even if she wasn't being forgotten about.

Many more examples and many more times, those familiar feelings haunted her over the years. She didn't know why, but she knew there was something wrong with her. There must be, or people wouldn't keep making her have that horrible feeling. And it was so horrible that she had to find a way to stop it from happening, but she couldn't think what to do. She didn't know what it was that made people treat her that way, so she couldn't try to fix whatever was wrong with her. She didn't know why they treated her that way, so she couldn't find a way to stop them from doing it. She was very unhappy.

That was when her subconscious mind stepped in. It had a few ideas and it wasn't sure if they would work, but it knew that it couldn't let her know what it was doing, because she was still quite young and not able to keep a secret. So it made a few changes of its own and watched to see if it was having the desired effect. It had learnt that people treated her differently when she was ill, and that, apart from the discomfort of the illness, she was happier when she was ill than when she was well. When she got better, people went back to their old ways and she felt that horrible old familiar feeling again.

So that was it. As long as she was ill, and took a long time to recover, those nasty feelings stayed away. If there was a good and effective treatment for whatever she had, it would have to not work quite so well for her. If there was anything going around, any infection, virus or bacteria, she would have to catch it. And her subconscious mind was in control of all that. That bit was easy to arrange. So it did.

Chris: *But was there really something wrong with her? Where had that idea first come from?*

Me: It hadn't crossed her mind until that day out shopping that December all those years ago. Sophie had long forgotten it along with the sadness of finding out that Santa wasn't a real person and that Mum and Dad had bought all those presents. But her subconscious mind hadn't forgotten it. It knew that Mum was loving and caring, and that she hadn't been too heavy at the time, so there must have been something wrong with her, and all those other times when she'd felt the same, people had 'put her down' in some way or other, so it wasn't just Mum that saw her that way.

But her subconscious didn't know, at that time, when she was only 5 years old, that she was bigger than her sister, heavier because she was taller even though she was thinner, and she didn't know that her mum wasn't as strong as her dad who was a builder and was used to carrying weights much heavier than her little chubby sister. And with that extra perspective, her subconscious mind was able to reassess that 'put-down' and that old familiar feeling strangely went away from that cold December day. There wasn't anything wrong with her, she was just older, taller and therefore heavier – her mum was smaller, did an office job, and had recently recovered from flu. Mum didn't mean it was Sophie's fault in any way. It wasn't anyone's fault – it was just how it was.

With that new, clearer and more comfortable explanation, that suspicion that there was something wrong with her could be re-written by her subconscious mind. And without that suspicion, all those other times when she'd felt that horrible feeling, they didn't look quite the same as they had before. Steadily, her subconscious mind began to see that there wasn't anything wrong with her, that she didn't need to feel that way, that she didn't need to expect to be treated that way, so she didn't need to be so ill, so often ill, so resistant to the best medical care and treatment.

Chris: *I'm beginning to see it a bit more clearly now, and I'm considering some treatment for my fear of driving. Then, if that goes well, I might just let you work on my peanut allergy.*

Me: I thought that was your friend.

Chris: *No it's me – and it's very scary, so if there's a chance of a cure, I would really want to give it a try. But I haven't made up my mind yet. If I do want treatment, I'd like to start with the more obviously psychological symptom first, but I need to give it some thought and discuss it with my family.*

I have another problem too, but I'm even more scared about having that one treated.

Me: If you want to tell me about it, and what it is you're scared about, I might be able to help.

Chris: *Ok. They call it O.C.D. Obsessive Compulsive Disorder. Have you heard of it?*

Me: Yes, but like all diagnoses, it can vary between patients. Tell me how it affects you.

Chris: *I have to check everything 10 times over. Everything has to be spotlessly clean and I need to clean and tidy up for hours after anything has been touched or moved or disturbed. And it's wearing me out.*

Me: I can imagine it would. So tell me what you are scared about.

Chris: *If I have treatment, then I don't know how I'll manage to live afterwards. It's such a big part of my life and I've lived with it for so long, so I can't imagine doing anything different – and not checking, not cleaning and tidying, that scares me. I don't know why, but it's terrifying. I only relax when I'm doing all that stuff. I'm physically exhausted but fairly relaxed mentally. When I try not to do it, like when I had some treatment a few years ago and they said I had to try, I was beside myself.*

Me: Well as you know, LCH is different. There's no need to try to do anything that you don't want to.

Chris: *That's part of my fear. In a way, I feel fortunate that it didn't work. LCH sounds so powerful and effective, I'm scared I will suddenly find all my habits and routines gone, and I don't know how, or even who I'll be without them.*

Me: I can understand that. You need to know that when treatment is successfully completed, the symptom, the compulsion fades away without any effort or fear. And it's likely to happen at a rate that you'll be able to get used to. The subconscious mind manages any changes it makes. It causes symptoms to be replaced gradually with healthier alternatives.

Chris: *I detect one of your stories brewing...*

Me: No it's a Blue Peter moment – here's one I made earlier.

Colin has a table with a leg that got broken one day when he fell against it after a heavy session down the pub. The rest of the table is ok. Buying a new table is out of the question for him – he can't afford it.

All he has available is some strong tape to wrap around the damaged leg. That makes the table functional up to a point. It will hold some weight – not as much as when it was sound – but enough to hold the essentials – and he has to handle it a bit gently, move it with care and only if absolutely necessary.

Colin eventually gets a bit fed up with this situation – he wants his fully functioning, strong and sturdy table back – so he decides to go to the table-leg-removers.

The table-leg-remover says "No worries, Colin, we can sort this for you. Leave it with us for a few days, and by the time we're done, all traces of that broken leg will be gone – completely. We've got this chain-saw that is really good at doing a clean and thorough job of removing table legs – whatever is wrong with them, whether they're broken or rotten or just a bit wonky, this chain-saw will remove them properly. What's more, we have this other machine that will turn the damaged wood into sawdust so that that damaged leg can never be re-fitted onto your table. Your table will never again have that damaged, wonky leg, wrapped around with tape, that leaves you worrying every day whether it will collapse"

Colin is most impressed. He leaves his table with the table-leg-removers, and a few days later he comes back to find that everything that he was promised has been done. All traces of his damaged table leg are gone. He happily and proudly takes his well-repaired table back home and decides he'll try it out straight away. It's nearly tea-time so he pictures himself sitting at his posh and well repaired table, eating his meal.

That's when he realises that the subject of replacing that leg had somehow never come up. Although it was broken and frail and needed strong tape to hold it together, it was, up to a point, doing its job. If he didn't put much on the table, and didn't move the table about much, it served all his essential needs. But now his table

wouldn't stand up at all. He didn't know what
to do. He only knew about table-leg-removers.
He didn't know of any table-leg-fitters. So he
sat on the floor and swore a bit.

Chris: *That's it. That's what I'm frightened of. I don't
know anything about replacement table legs.
I've never even heard of them. I can't picture
what such a thing might look like, never mind
having any idea where I might get one and how
I'd be able to get it fixed on. I can't imagine life
without my OCD and my cleaning so I won't be
leaving my table with the leg-removers.*

Me: Remember that the subconscious mind is our
best friend, our big sister, our mum and our
personal assistant. She won't take away that
leg until she's sure we can manage without it.
She doesn't let that scab fall off until the skin
beneath it has healed.

Chris: *And if we pick it off early, she gives us another
one to take its place.*

Me: That's right. And if we recover from the flu
symptoms but aren't fully fighting fit yet, she
makes us tired and uninspired so we continue to
rest until we've recharged our batteries again.

Chris: *So she'll make those changes happen at a rate
that I can adapt to, is that right?*

Me: Yes, she might encourage you to stretch yourself
a bit and venture out of your comfortable corner,
but not to enter the triathlon until you're trained
and are fit enough.

Chris: *Ok, I'll think it over and see how I get on with my driving first. I'm more relaxed about that one. I don't need to drive so I can have treatment for that and then decide about the other ones after that.*

Me: Good idea.

A friend of my friends

Alex has a history of childhood abuse and now, as an adult, has severe drug addiction.

Alex: *I want to be free of my addiction. I want to live a normal, happy life. Pat and Chris have both been helping me with the kids and with getting myself a bit healthier, eating better and looking after myself – but whenever I start making some real progress, it always seems to get sabotaged by my drug addiction. They said you might be able to help me.*

Me: I might. You clearly want help. You've been trying to make things better – and your motivation is a crucial part of getting the best result from treatment.

Alex: *But surely someone with my kind of background must be too damaged to ever be properly healthy?*

Me: You suffered as a child and you're still suffering now?

Alex: *Yes!*

Me: The fact that you ask that question tells me that even though you don't expect a better life, you want it and you know you deserve it.

Alex: In one way, yes you're right, but there's a part of
me that wonders if I'm really so bad, deep down,
through and through, that those people who
hurt me were right all along – that they were just
giving me what I deserved. If I didn't deserve it,
why did they pick on me?

Me: Do you want to be bad, to hurt people, to cause
harm?

Alex: No! But maybe that's my nature – and as much
as I fight it, it will just keep on coming through.
If I'm dirty, then any perfume I put on will only
hide it for a while. If the house is damp, then air-
fresheners will only give an illusion that the air is
fresh. Maybe it's just how I am.

Me: You're telling me you want to be good but you
worry that you might be bad, so I believe you
deserve all the help you can get. If you find
yourself causing harm, however hard you try, then
I believe it's help, not punishment, that you need.

Alex: So how could you help me? Nothing has worked
up to now. I've had counselling and I've got a
social worker who tries to keep me straight, but
I keep slipping back every time.

Me: If anyone feels bad and beats themselves up over
something they've done, or even everything they
do, then there's got to be a contradiction there.
If you truly were bad and truly deserved to be
punished, you wouldn't be worrying about the
harm you'd caused, the people you'd hurt and
accepting your punishment as deserved. You'd be

out there making sure you didn't get caught –
you'd be making sure you got the first punch in.

If you intended to cause harm, you caused harm
and you were happy, your only concern would
be to evade punishment – happy if someone
else got the blame instead of you, maybe even
framing someone else.

None of that applies to you, does it?

Alex: No!

  Me: So if you've caused harm, it was accidentally done,
innocently done, or maybe you were backed into a
corner and it was your only means of survival.

Alex: *Yes – all of those!*

  Me: Ok so you need help, support and guidance, not
punishment, right?

Alex: *Yes!*

  Me: And this addiction is a big part of what's getting
in your way. Where did it come from?

Alex: *Well initially, I tried it out of curiosity, and
someone made it sound fun and exciting – and
now it's in my system – it's a physical addiction.
The withdrawal symptoms are dangerous.*

  Me: Ok but with medical assistance, people have
managed that withdrawal and got over it,
haven't they?

Alex: *Yes but they're strong and I'm not.*

  Me: I have to disagree. The life that you've been
living has been anything but easy. You've had it

rough and you're still surviving. You've been knocked down over and over – and picked yourself up again every time, right?

Alex: *Yes.*

Me: So you're strong too?

Alex: *Yes ok – but I don't feel strong. It feels like every time I try to change things, something gets in my way.*

Me: What kind of something?

Alex: *Life – circumstances.*

Me: Do you find yourself always walking into trouble however hard you try to stay clean?

Alex: *Yes I do.*

Me: So does it feel like you're accident-prone?

Alex: *Yes, something like that.*

Me: And from a purely rational point of view, just looking at the bare facts, is there actually any reason for that kind of thing to happen more to you than to anyone else?

Alex: *No, I suppose not – and it's not fair!*

Me: No, I agree and that's why I believe you deserve some help.

Alex: *Yes but how?*

Me: When we walk into trouble, there has to be something making our feet go in that direction – and if your feet are drawn towards trouble more

often that most people's, then that has to be
something to do with you, doesn't it?

Alex: *Well no – I could just be unlucky.*

Me: Ok – if you're unlucky, then I can't do anything
to help you. But if it's something within you,
then I probably can. So which would you prefer
it to be?

Alex: *Are you saying that you could help me stop
walking into trouble?*

Me: If you work with me, then yes, probably.

Alex: *Ok then I'd rather believe it's inside me. But that
would just be wishful thinking, wouldn't it?*

Me: I've been working and studying and developing
for years now in order to make as sure as
I possibly can that I don't waste anyone's time
or money, that I don't do any harm, and that
I don't raise false hopes - and I wouldn't be having
this conversation with you if I hadn't already
successfully treated a lot of people with conditions
just as puzzling and persistent as yours.

But I don't expect you to take that on trust.
I expect you to want to know what LCH is
all about, so you can decide for yourself if it's
something you can understand and trust.

Alex: *Pat and Chris have told me a few things, so
I have an idea about it already – and it makes
sense and sounds safe – but as I've told you,
I've been abused and I wonder if the damage
is already too deep to be fully corrected.*

Me: Many people struggle to give up smoking. Some say it's harder to come off tobacco than heroin, not because of the physical withdrawal but because it's so fully ingrained in the smoker's life. I treated someone using LCH because they had been smoking for about 40 years and were thoroughly sick of it, but couldn't stop. They'd tried everything, the gum, the patches, tablets from the doctor, anti-smoking clinics, everything.

After treatment, this person didn't want to smoke, hadn't smoked for a few weeks, but felt the need to test it out. Most people, even those who successfully treat smokers using traditional hypnotherapy suggestion, advise that a single cigarette is highly likely to re-kindle that addiction – that the addiction is lying there dormant and ready to spring back into life. This person wanted to know if the addiction was still there inside them.

They lit a cigarette and took a drag and disliked the taste. They took a second drag – wanting to give it a thorough test – and it tasted even worse. They wanted to be totally sure that it was gone so they took a third drag and couldn't continue. They disliked it so much that they stubbed it out, and as far as I know (up to date many months have passed since that test-smoke) they haven't wanted a cigarette and haven't felt any need to test it out any further. I imagine that's how a non-smoker would react to such a test.

I've treated people who have suffered from bulimia and have, for years, made themselves vomit several times a day. Following successful treatment, they've found that urge reducing in intensity and frequency until they've again had many months without their old most-unwelcome habit. One commented that they now found the idea of vomiting and of making themselves vomit as repulsive and as alien as they imagined most 'healthy' people found it. And that person had had the habit for many years with no concern or distaste for the actual process of purging – just a relief that the food had been removed before it could be absorbed.

People go to huge lengths to reduce weight. They try all the slimming diets, tablets from the doctor, surgery, gastric bands to reduce the capacity of the stomach. Many of these people are so obese that their life is seriously at risk as a result. And even if it doesn't kill them, it severely restricts their life, drastically reduces their chance of fun and happiness. So it might seem a minor concern compared to your drug addiction, but at that end of the scale, there are some similarities.

Alex: *No, I don't agree. The people that know I'm a user shun me in the street. I get called names and worse.*

Me: There are people so heavy that they are physically unable to leave their house. There was a program on TV years ago showing how, because the scales at the clinic had a limit that some people had exceeded, the people had to go to an industrial unit to be weighed on a platform designed for weighing the factory's products.

Alex: *Ok – but what has that got to do with me?*

Me: I've treated several people who have had a life-long battle with their weight, with food, with eating. They've beaten themselves up for eating a slice of bread or a potato believing they were bad for having given in to temptation and that they should have been satisfied with celery and an apple. They've gone out to the corner shop or the garage late at night for chocolate, and one finally came to me after she found herself rummaging through a rubbish bin to satisfy that craving.

Alex: *Yes it does sound serious.*

Me: People with cravings and habits like that have come back to me after treatment describing going to a restaurant, a special occasion, for a treat, and only having a simple main course, no starter or dessert, and not even finishing what was on their plate. That was all they wanted and they enjoyed the evening. Someone else took a couple of crisps from someone else's pack when offered and didn't then feel any urge to get a bag for themselves. Another took a small slice of birthday cake at a party and noticed afterwards that they'd only had a couple of bites and left the rest.

Alex: *That sounds like hard work.*

Me: No, these were all experiences that the people had when they weren't trying. They weren't dieting, just being guided by what they wanted – and what they wanted was totally different from the kind of food and the quantity of food they'd wanted before.

Alex: *So you've treated people with serious conditions and you've had some successes. I'm with you so far, but I don't really understand what LCH is about except that it looks for the underlying cause. I've been abused and I don't want to talk about it any more. They made me do all that at the police station, in court and with that therapist. I don't want to go through all that again.*

Me: I don't need you to. LCH doesn't rely on any of that kind of work.

Alex: *So how does it work?*

Me: Imagine a plant pot with some fresh rich soil in it. It's getting the right amount of water and sunshine and plant food. If there's no seed in that soil, nothing will grow however much it's nurtured.

Alex: *Ok, but what's that got to do with me?*

Me: Some people would suggest that the kind of childhood you've had would be a fertile soil for problems like addictions, anxiety, low self-esteem as an adult. So they'd suggest something like your drug addiction is an inevitable consequence of damage suffered as a child.

Alex: *And they might be right.*

Me: Some people have backgrounds like yours and, with help and support and guidance, they go on to live happy, healthy and productive lives. They get the help they need and eventually put it all behind them and live how they want to. There are many of them who have financed their happier future from their autobiographies telling uplifting stories of survival against the odds.

Alex: *How can they do that?*

Me: I believe that the people who can turn things round in that way had no seed in their plant pot in the first place. I believe that the therapy that you had, and any support and help you've received along the way, has failed to help you move on because there was a seed in your plant pot – and all that childhood pain was what made it grow into a poisonous plant that is now keeping you unhealthy and unhappy.

Alex: *Pat and Chris told me some of your stories. Is that seed one of those incidents that was misunderstood?*

Me: Yes and it's extremely likely to have absolutely nothing to do with any of those painful memories – and even if there's some kind of connection, I don't need you to remember anything, to re-experience anything, to re-live anything at all. In fact, treatment is a lot quicker and easier if you allow me to guide you on how to leave me to do my job while you go off and daydream.

Alex: *I can certainly do that easily enough! And it sounds like I have nothing to lose. Dad says he'll pay for my treatment and will look after the kids for me while I see you, but will I be able to do it? What if I'm the one it doesn't work for? You only said*

*'probably' so it can't work for everyone – what if
I'm the one that can't do it?*

Me: You have those worries because they go together
with all that you've described to me, and until
we fix the underlying cause, you'll be likely to
continue to worry about it – but I'm not worried.
I'll guide you through it step by step, and I'm
confident you'll get on ok.

So you can worry if you want to, and you can let
me get on with my work and we can both watch
those worries fade way.

LCH – history and training

As Alex went away to think it over, Pat came back, and as I might have predicted, had even more questions for me.

Pat: *Where did LCH come from? Who invented it? Why is it called Lesserian?*

Me: David Lesser started this amazing journey with his work doing therapeutic massage. It wasn't long before he began to see a clear connection between the body and the mind as a result of his hands-on treatment of his patients. The loosening of tight muscles seemed to cause some letting go of mental, psychological difficulties.

His enquiring mind soon turned that connection around and asked it some questions. If what you do to the body can affect the mind, then can what you do the mind affect the body?

His own work with hypnosis and hypnotherapy provided a few clues and lit up a few corridors with a few doors leading from them, and my broad-brush mental picture of the scenario is that he found himself in some very interesting and therapeutically productive rooms. To him it was obvious. You just had to open that door.

Pat: *Which door?*

Me: That one, the obvious one, the only one.

Pat: *Well it's not obvious to me.*

Me: Not to me either, and this is really my own interpretation of various snippets of information that I've picked up along the way, but in my opinion, it was only obvious to David himself.

Pat: *You're being incredibly vague. Can you be more specific?*

Me: I can – but stay with me for a while, because I think it will make more sense to you if I explain in my own way.

Pat: *Ok. Go on.*

Me: My main hobby is a partner dance called Lindy Hop. I go to classes and workshops and dance my socks off – and it's so much fun to learn and develop and stretch into. Some people dance so naturally, so easily, find themselves creating moves that look so exciting that we all want to have a go. And some of those talented people set up classes and start to teach. And it's only when you start trying to explain that you learn that explaining what you just did automatically is quite a bit more tricky that you first thought.

If it's easy for me, then I just need to show you and it'll be easy for you too, right?

Pat: *Not for me – and I've seen how hard they work on Strictly Come Dancing, so I think it's not just me.*

Me: Not for me either! I can't get it just by watching.
I need help. I need to see it broken down into steps
and those steps explained in a way that makes
sense to my way of absorbing and interpreting
information. The steps you break it down into can
be linear, chronological, functional or some other
slicing direction. In dancing terms, you can break
down a move that takes 8 beats of the music into
what you do on beats 1-4, then what you do on
beats 5-8. And if that's not enough, you can break
it down into beats 1-2, 3-4, 5-6, 7-8. And so on.
And then you'd need to join up those parts again -
how beat 4 flows into beat 5 And eventually,
having identified small steps so simple that all the
class have mastered them, and having connected
each pairing of small steps with its adjacent small
steps and all the class have got that too, you have
a whole sequence and all can do it.

But it doesn't look quite the same as when the
teachers dance it. And to me, it doesn't feel right
either. It doesn't actually work for me. I'm not a
performer. I dance for how it feels to me, and
as this is a partner dance, I dance to enjoy that
musical conversation with my partner. And I still
can't get it.

So they analyze even further what they are doing
and how they are doing it.

They see that the shape they are making is different
from ours. So how are they achieving that shape?
Lindy Hop is a fun, playful, exciting dance, and
when you examine what processes are involved in

making it flow, you see that it makes use of the laws of physics. In order to give moves some dynamics, you need to create a rubber-band effect. You need to use stretch and compression. It's based on 'lead and follow' where the leader starts a musical conversation and the follower replies.

If the only connection between the leader and the follower is that the leader's left hand is holding the follower's right hand, then if the leader's dancing is going to have any chance of steering the follower's direction and driving the follower's pace, then the leader and follower need to connect their own hand to their own arm, to their own body so that a slight movement in the leader's body, a change of direction, a lateral rotation, a sudden braking force are all transmitted to the follower's body in the form of a twist, a turn, a slide, a jump.

So clearly, you can't teach all that's required to create that conversation, that message transfer, all that resulting look and feel, if you divide the move into beats. You have to find other ways to slice it up. You need to create exercises that develop the stretching and compression, that foster that connection between the hand and arm and body, that encourage the leader to let his own dancing create the movement rather than stand still and steer his follower with his arms, that helps the follower to behave like a shopping trolley out in space. The follower needs to go in the direction she's sent and to continue going until stopped or redirected. Those exercises are practiced over and over until they become automatic. If you have to think about it, then it will be awkward and too slow.

Try walking on the spot and moving opposing arms. Try just walking down the street and then just noticing what your arms are doing. If we leave them to it, they do it perfectly well. If we try to take over, it often seems to goes wrong.

So the best teachers of Lindy Hop are those who can see what they are doing, what is causing something to work, what needs to become automatic, what specifically needs to be practiced. They can also look at what the dancers in their class are doing and devise some exercises to help replace any automatic but unproductive habits with ones that will make the dance flow.

Pat: *I really get that about dancing because of all the examples they show on the TV, but what has that got to do with LCH?*

Me: David Lesser was able to treat his patients, moving instinctively down the right corridor into the right room, striding confidently to that desk drawer and finding that all-important clue to unlock the patient's fear, addiction, symptom, condition. But as it was so obvious to him, he maybe didn't see how it could not be obvious to others.

So it took another pair of eyes to start to observe, analyze, dissect and begin to explain some of the steps that were only obvious to David himself. His daughter, Helen, decided to join him in his chosen profession in 1982, attended his training course and started treating patients. Maybe some of David's instincts were inherited and she was able to also instinctively open the right doors without knowing exactly how she knew which were the right doors. She had moved on from where David was because, unlike him, she could see that there were other doors that, based on her training, would have been logical alternatives.

But to pass it on to other people who hadn't inherited that same instinct, and maybe to check if some of those other doors were, in fact, just as valuable and viable, she started to analyze a bit more deeply.

This process went on and on for years. It's still going on. She finds new ways to explain, new images to help switch on the various light-bulbs in the heads of the students. She even created a whole new framework that, when followed rigorously, makes a successful outcome more reliable, more frequently attained.

I was fortunate enough to arrive after she created that framework, and I know that it feels vital to me that it is there to guide me through the treatment.

Small steps

Pat: *I understand so much from your pictures and stories, and I'm really keen to enrol on the training course, but I'm nervous that I won't be up to the challenge. Can you help me with that?*

Me: It's not unusual to be nervous about a new project and to wonder if we'll be able to do something we've never tried before, so I felt exactly the same and might just be able to offer you some ideas to consider and try out.

All the way through my journey from hearing about LCH to where I am now as a qualified and experienced therapist, with aims and plans to go further along that path, become more efficient in what I do and spread the word about LCH even further, I've occasionally stared at a brick wall over 10 feet high, knowing that where I was aiming to reach was beyond it. At first, I would stand and look at it in despair, in the middle of the night, immobilised and not knowing what to do. But then the beginnings of some daylight - dawn was breaking - showed me some hand and foot holes in the wall. I went to the gym, did some exercises and developed some strength in my fingers and toes and overcame that particular personal hurdle.

And then, I would notice a parallel track which could be navigated fairly easily by a giant, 3 steps, each 3ft high that I could scramble up with some help from a nearby traveller. I'd get there, but I'd arrive exhausted and with grazed knees.

Then the full light of day would illuminate yet another route. It was a set of stairs, each no more than 6 inches high, and I could take them one at a time, could stop and rest, pretending I was admiring the view whenever I was tired - and could reach that destination without working up a sweat, without even scuffing my shoes.

Pat: *So what causes the light to come on?*

Me: Nature does it. The laws of physics, gravity, the rotation of the earth as it travels along its regular orbit of the sun brings new light every single day.

Pat: *Oh for goodness sake! I worry about you sometimes! The lights in your head, the navigable paths, the stepping stones, the understanding and the ideas, where do they all come from?*

Me: I rely on the subconscious mind - my personal assistant and my best friend. If I ask them, and if they can help, and if they believes that what I'm asking for is right for me, then they will switch the lights on for me, one at a time so my eyes can adjust, and hold my hand if the path is a bit rocky and steep.

I tell them what I want to do, what I'm trying to achieve, what I would like to happen – and then I trust them to do their job. I leave them to it like

I might leave the bread-machine and the slow-cooker on so that, after a hard day's work, there's a tasty and nutritious meal of stew and crusty wholemeal all ready to serve up.

Pat: *How do you do that?*

Me: Whenever I find that I haven't got a clue how to complete a particular task, I mentally ask for some help and then I rely on them to bring it to me. I know that some idea will come along, some time in the next few hours or days, and that will point me towards some smaller steps, some other path, someone or something that can help me.

Pat: *And has that always worked for you?*

Me: Not always. Sometimes I found that I needed to work really hard but still hardly made any progress. I wasn't getting the results I expected so the first thing to check on was whether I was doing all the right things in all the right ways. I was working on the Diploma, repeated the Practical Course as a refresher and worked intensively with my supervisor. She and I looked in detail at various aspects of my work until she was able to confirm that I was doing enough of the right things to be getting much better results than I had been getting.

Pat: *So what did you do?*

Me: I gave myself the same advice as I would give a potential patient. I found myself an LCH therapist.

My treatment

Pat: *Can you tell me this in detail, then? Do you mind other people knowing? Chris is here too. Will you tell us both?*

Me: Yes this bit is all factual. Nothing has been amended. It's true and correct and complete as far as I remember. So here, finally, is some information I'm allowed to give. I give myself permission to give this confidential information – the patient was me. Hardly statistically significant, purely anecdotal – but maybe, just maybe there's some understanding to be gained from it, some clue as to what is happening when we get sick, ill, when the body goes out of balance in some way.

At the age of 55, I went to the doctor with a symptom which is, apparently, cause for much concern in a woman of my age. The doctor arranged an urgent appointment at the local hospital's PMB department - for the investigation of Post-Menopausal Bleeding. Within 2 weeks, I was there, having various tests.

The attitude and manner of the staff of that department left me puzzled. I was asked how I was. I replied that I was fine. One member of staff gave me a kind of concerned look and added for me, "As well as can be expected?" They were treating me with kid gloves. They had boxes of tissues handy. The treatment was preceded and followed with an interview, one-to-one, with a very sympathetic nurse who, beforehand, explained what the tests would involve, and afterwards, what the tests had shown up, and what they advised should be the next steps.

I later did some reading on the internet and found recommendations for medical practitioners along the lines that post-menopausal bleeding was to be assumed to be cancerous until proved otherwise. The reactions from the hospital staff made much more sense after that. They probably assumed I'd already done that research before my appointment, or that that message had filtered through to me via the doctor and the speed of my referral.

It seemed that the main concern was that the ultrasound had shown up a thickening of the lining of the womb. This was a symptom that needed to be fully and urgently checked out. Delay could result in more radical treatment becoming necessary. It could be a benign symptom, in which case, no treatment would be needed, but they advised an urgent biopsy, which involved a surgical procedure under general anaesthetic – and predicted that this would happen within the next 2 or 3 weeks.

At this point, I started to sit up and take a lot more notice. It had almost passed me by, just on the edge of my awareness that the first appointment had been within two weeks. I had heard of lengthy waiting lists, and lengthy waits to get on those lengthy lists and then lengthy waits to reach the top. But I'd been seen for tests within 2 weeks and was expecting to have an operation within 4 or 5 weeks of my original GP appointment.

But I wanted time to think. I had questions spinning around my head. I asked for time to explore other options – but I wanted to take a safe route, so I also asked for some idea of the expected consequences of any delay. I wanted time to go to an LCH therapist so that she could ask my subconscious mind why this symptom was happening and follow clues back to the underlying cause with a view to correcting any mistaken information.

The nurse seemed amazed. She'd probably never had such a reaction before. She explained that a delay could mean the difference between needing chemotherapy - or the less-invasive radiotherapy, and between more or less radical surgery. But she was prepared to accept my suggestion that I take a couple of months to explore the hypnotherapy option and then repeat the ultrasound test.

And this is exactly what happened. I went for a number of sessions with a very experienced therapist, one with more than 20 years experience as a full-time practitioner. After a number of weekly sessions, she told me that my subconscious had indicated that the symptom was no longer needed and was being disposed of.

About 3 weeks after that, I attended for the repeat
ultra-sound test. I have to admit to being nervous.
I knew what the likely consequences were for me if
the test results were the same as before or worse. I
knew that the biopsy would then be needed and that
the results could mean that I would need extensive
cancer treatment – and that treatment might not be
totally successful. It was a big day for me.

I had my repeat ultrasound and then had my
interview with the same nurse as I had seen the
previous time. She didn't keep me in suspense for
long. She said that the results were much better
now, that the thickness of the lining of my womb
was now within normal limits, that they were not
now recommending the surgical procedure. In
fact, they weren't even recommending a repeat test
in a few months time. They were discharging me!

She said something along the lines of, "maybe
it was the hypnotherapy, maybe it was your
hormones, who knows, but whatever caused it,
the news is good."

As I walked out of the hospital, the sun was
shining, the birds were singing, and I was walking
on a cushion of air. I could hardly wait to get home
to ring my therapist with the news. She and I were
both delighted.

The reason why I left this until the last is to make
sure that you have the best chance of seeing this
information in perspective. There is no way
I would ever recommend anyone else to do what
I did. At times I can't quite believe it myself. I also

know that there is no 'happily ever after' in real life. There is no knowing what I should have done, whether I did the right thing, whether I took an unnecessary risk - whether I'm still taking one.

I'm like the scientist who believes so strongly in the therapy I'm providing that I make my own mind up, make my own decisions, go with what feels right for me. I'm an adult, and as far as I know, of sound mind - although based on what I've just described, others may disagree, and I respect their opinion. I feel free to go where my heart and subconscious mind seem to be guiding me.

But maybe, just maybe, this causes someone, somewhere to wonder if there's something worth researching into, some possibility that my subconscious mind did actually change what was possibly a pre-cancerous, or even already cancerous condition back into a healthy one because someone talked to her, to Amy, and asked her some questions, dozens, hundreds of questions and then suggested that some information might have been misunderstood and might benefit from a reinterpretation.

Maybe, just maybe....

Pat: *And what could have caused this?*

Me: I found that a memory came back to me after one of my treatment sessions. I don't know for sure if this was the cause or just a part of it, but it certainly had all the right ingredients that would cause an LCH therapist to investigate it fully.

I was about 4 yrs old at the time - and that's a guess because I can remember looking up at the sideboard and having to reach up to it, and at much more than 4 years old, I would have been tall enough not to have had to reach up. I went into the front room and noticed something new on the sideboard. It was a model boat, maybe about 12 inches long. I picked it up with the curiosity of a young child. It was the finished article of what my elder brother, then about 9 years old, had been spending so much time and attention on over the previous few months. As I lifted it off, its stand or base fell to the floor.

I knew that my brother had made it and thought he had forgotten to glue it to the base. I thought it was an ornament that the base was a part of – and the glue was there on the sideboard, next to boat and its base.

I was excited to think that I could help, I wanted to help and thought I'd found a good way to pay back all that my elder brother had done for me. I figured that if I glued the boat to the base, no-one would ever know that my brother had forgotten to do that bit and I would have helped him. I was very fond of and proud of my older brother and felt good that I had found a way to help him.

My brother had taken months to build the boat from a kit, a task which took patience and hours of delicate work for a 9 year old. That much I knew. But what I didn't know was that he had been looking forward to his first opportunity of sailing it on the park lake. Now, because of my 'helpfulness', it wouldn't sail because it was fixed to its base.

I was in the front room on my own and overheard raised voices. My brother was saying to Mum "Look what she's done, she's ruined it! I'll break her neck. I'll kill her.' Such graphic expressions were common in the household. Dad in temper would often say what he would do to whoever had crossed him and Aunty would explain in detail what the bogeyman in the park would do if he caught me and what would happen if I fell off the swing in the park – that it would crack my skull open. This was the 1950's - no-one paid too much attention to that kind of wording.

But the anger, frustration and blame were clear messages. It seemed, to my 4 year old ears, like Mum was having to physically restrain my brother from entering the room I was in and carrying out his deadly threats.

Mum was trying to offer the voice of reason. "She didn't mean to do it, she was only trying to help, she didn't know you wanted to sail it".

My brother, at 9 years old, was already a caring and nurturing big brother. He would take me with him on trips to local parks and other kid-friendly places, which in the 1950's included a lot more than it does today. But all of that went out of the window because he was too consumed with his frustration that his months of patient and careful work was now ruined. In the heat of the moment, he said: "Well she should have known! It's a boat! She's stupid!"

Mum's praise "only trying to help" had less credence than my brother's "she should have known – she's stupid", because Mum always said nice things to and about me and because Mum never managed to be subtle in her attempts to let me win in games and competitions. I had already, even at that tender age, begun to dismiss Mum's comments as being what Mum always said. My brother, on the other hand, had always spoken the truth as far as I knew up to then.

That was a tiny nudge off the happy healthy path that I, and everyone else in the world, started out on. Other experiences confirmed my stupidity with little or no evidence that would stand up on its own in court. Expressions like 'give a dog a bad name' and 'there's no smoke without fire' had been influencing the verdict. My subconscious mind had gradually taken less and less convincing that that next event had provided even more damning confirmation that I was in fact stupid!

And I can be more comfortable now with any symptom or condition or issue that I get. I don't need to learn that it's physical, detectable scientifically. As a therapist, I can tell my patients that I've had treatment for conditions similar to the ones I also treat, and that my treatment isn't yet complete because I presented my therapist with a huge shopping list and she's steadily working her way through it.

I'm comfortable with this, mentally, because I see the 'mind that it's all in' as someone connected to me, but not actually me. The part of me that I'm aware of, that I can control and steer and feel responsible or accountable for, isn't the part that creates symptoms, conditions and issues. I can retain my self-esteem as an intelligent person and a therapist if I become ill or uncomfortable or distressed. I simply go to my specialist and she invariably finds that there's a perfectly plausible reason based on some erroneous information – and alone, I would be powerless to fix it.

I can now, with the wonderful gift of hindsight, see the reason why I had managed to go through various courses being the only person around at the time that expected me to fail each type of assessment. I seemed quite incapable of rational appraisal of my academic history, totally oblivious to previous high grades, and entered every exam convinced I would fail.

I chivvied myself along with "if I give it my best, it might just make the difference between a fail and a scraped pass", and in the case of my degree in Economics from Lancaster University, found to my amazement several months later that it had resulted in an Upper Second Class Honours that had even caused some discussion among the assessors as to whether my submissions warranted a viva voce with the possible outcome of a conversion to a First. It wasn't just a 2.1, it was a good 2.1!!!

And I was also being treated for a food allergy
which is now a thing of the past, a bony spur
on one of the joints of the little finger of my left
hand, which is also now gone – as well as various
issues around my lack of self-confidence, my lack
of belief in my ability to succeed, maybe even a
fear of success that kept me in the background,
hardly able to open my mouth to speak.

Chris: *You should write a book about it!*

Me: Hmmmm...

Note from the author:

This book has been completed but I see the subject itself, everything to do with my study of LCH and the subconscious mind as work in progress. I welcome any feedback, any ideas or questions or comments raised for you by this book and will take any appropriate communications into account in my future written work – maintaining your confidentiality just as I have with my patients' stories.

If you want more information about treatment or training, or if you wish to send me any feedback of your own, you will find my contact details via my website www.curativehypnotherapyyork.co.uk and the training college website is www.lesserian.co.uk

Cheers! – Salud! – Santé! – Salute! - Je via sano!

Mary Ratcliffe